POLITICAL SOCIOLOGY AND
THE PEOPLE'S HEALTH

Small Books, Big Ideas in Population Health
Series Editor
Nancy Krieger

POLITICAL SOCIOLOGY AND THE PEOPLE'S HEALTH

Jason Beckfield
PROFESSOR AND CHAIR OF
SOCIOLOGY
HARVARD UNIVERSITY
ASSOCIATE DIRECTOR OF
THE HARVARD CENTER FOR
POPULATION AND DEVELOPMENT
STUDIES

OXFORD
UNIVERSITY PRESS

Oxford University Press is a department of the University of Oxford. It furthers
the University's objective of excellence in research, scholarship, and education
by publishing worldwide. Oxford is a registered trade mark of Oxford University
Press in the UK and certain other countries.

Published in the United States of America by Oxford University Press
198 Madison Avenue, New York, NY 10016, United States of America.

© Oxford University Press 2018

CIP data is on file at the Library of Congress
ISBN 978-0-19-049247-2

9 8 7 6 5 4 3 2 1

Printed by Sheridan Books, Inc., United States of America

Oxford University Press is not responsible for any websites (or their content) referred to in this book
that are not owned or controlled by the publisher.

CONTENTS

FOREWORD
For the People's Health—Why this Book Series
of Small Books with Big Ideas

Nancy Krieger

Dialogue. Allies. Critical Thinking.
And: Adversaries

Several years ago, when I first conceived of this series of small books
with big ideas to expand social epidemiology's contributions to
the ongoing collective quest for health equity, I knew that more
critical dialogue was needed—both within the discipline and with
allied disciplines, inside and outside the field of public health.
Concise texts provide an ideal forum in which to present this type
of critical thinking: provocative, probing, longer than a journal article, shorter than a tome, affordable, and accessible for assigning
as reading material for academic courses. The point of this series is
to make sharp ideas attractively available, motivated by the urgent
need for both critical thinking and action for the people's health.

Why? Three reasons.

The first reason, internal to the field, is that as a discipline
matures, it risks becoming set in its ways.[1,2] Founding channels of
initial inquiry deepen, often with little impetus for cross-irrigation,

and lines of debate get hardened, with arguments often circling round and round, rather than advancing.[1,2] Although the roots of social epidemiology can readily be traced back to the mid-19th century CE, to the rise of the field of public health and the health impacts of ravenously expanding industrial capitalism and dramatic expansions of global commerce and colonial rule,[3,4] nevertheless its first textbooks are progeny of the early 21st century.[3,5–13] It is thus timely to revisit the field's ideas, methods, and evidence, and to search out allies who can both inform the ideas that feed the hypotheses and data that social epidemiologists analyze and interpret, and also translate our field's findings into actionable steps for reducing health inequities and improving population health. Among the initial array of topics to be addressed in this series are connections between social epidemiology and diverse disciplines (e.g., political sociology, Latin American social medicine), issues (e.g., climate change, causal inference), and mechanisms (e.g., epigenetics)—and the list will expand.

A second reason is that fast-moving transformations—such as global climate change—are threatening the well-being of life on this planet in truly new and potentially catastrophic ways.[3,4,14–16] Posing challenges of a different sort is the increasingly rapid expansion of scales—from macro to micro—for data acquisition and analysis, from Big Data to the nanoscale.[17–20] A discipline's ideas, as well as methods, need not only keep up with the pace of change, but also, by dint of hard thinking grounded in empirical reality, anticipate what may soon unfold—and this again requires conceptually working with allies both in and outside of social epidemiology. Such collective engagement is an imperative for fields concerned with the prevention of preventable suffering, and inequities in such suffering—i.e., the very mission at the heart of social epidemiology.[3]

The third reason is that social epidemiology, as a discipline, needs to be clear on who and what are the adversaries that stand in the way of eradicating health inequities.[3,4] It is not enough, for example, to provide empirical evidence that, say, egalitarian and environmentally sustainable policies promote both health equity and population health. After all, at one level, such evidence should be in the proverbial American "Mom and apple pie" category of phenomena: who could possibly oppose such a seemingly beneficent and anodyne recommendation?

Except that clearly many can and do—because if the arguments for health equity were as compelling as many in social epidemiology would like to believe, all of us on this planet would be living in a very different, healthier, and more equitable world, one not imperiled by environmental degradation, climate change, and the avaricious private accumulation of more and more wealth by an ever smaller portion of the world's people, and its effect on local, national, and global governance and population health.[3,4,14–16,18,21] In January 2018, Oxfam reported:[21]

> Last year saw the biggest increase in the number of billionaires in history, with one more billionaire every two days. There are now 2,043 dollar billionaires worldwide. Nine out of 10 are men. Billionaires also saw a huge increase in their wealth. This increase was enough to end extreme poverty seven times over. Eighty-two percent of all of the growth in global wealth in the last year went to the top 1%, whereas the bottom 50% saw no increase at all.

This concentration of wealth has been accelerating since the 1980s,[21–23] a legacy of the post-1980 onslaught of neoliberal reforms, launched in reaction to the gains of the 1960s and 1970s against colonial rule and, in my country (the United States), gains in civil rights and economic justice.[3,4,23,24]

In the United States, as I write this introduction in February 2018, we confront a federal administration intent on dismantling environmental regulations and instead protecting and expanding the fossil fuel industries; slashing taxes and regulations for corporations and shrinking taxes for wealthy households, while decimating agencies and funding for social programs that help people live healthier lives; undercutting civil rights and attacking independent journalism, the rule of law, and scientific evidence; intensifying anti-immigrant policies and attacks on reproductive and sexual rights and health—all policies bolstered by a president whose endless tweets are a unique brand of ceaseless demagoguery, falsehoods, racism, misogyny, and disdain for actual knowledge.[23–27] As I have written elsewhere, the Trump administration appears to have a death wish when it comes to public health.[27] To make a difference, we in public health, including social epidemiology, need to be explicit about naming who and what harms the people's health, so as to promote accountability and alliances to galvanize change.

I am thus especially happy that the first book in this new series is Jason Beckfield's *Political Sociology and the People's Health*.[28] It could not be more timely. Beckfield cogently and concisely argues, in the book's allotted three chapters, what political sociology can contribute to social epidemiology, in terms of theories, constructs, measures, and methods, while also exploring how social epidemiology can help political sociology sharpen its own sets of ideas, methods, and evidence, drawing on our field's ideas about embodiment, populations, distributions, and etiologic period. He introduces social epidemiologists to clear frameworks, vocabularies, and approaches to conceptualizing and measuring what, in social epidemiology, are often loosely defined sets of phenomena variously grouped into the umbrella category of "social determinants of health." He likewise synthesizes the evidence on how and why political-social phenomena, at multiple levels, drive both on-average population health and health inequities, including inequities in relation to nationality, social class, gender, racism, religion, and sexuality. The exposition is lucid. Moreover, pointing to enormous gaps in evidence, Beckfield opens up a rich research agenda that is bound to foment productive inquiries and greater awareness of the political-social institutions and "rules of the game" that advocates for the people's health must challenge and change. Let the dialogue and debates begin!—so as to shore up the critical intellectual tools, arguments, and evidence needed in the collective fight to create conditions which ensure that all people can live dignified healthy lives in a sustainable manner on our shared and precious planet.

REFERENCES

1. Frodeman, R., Klein, J. T., & Pacheco, R. C. S. (eds.). (2017). *The Oxford Handbook of Interdisciplinarity*. 2nd ed. New York: Oxford University Press.
2. Ziman, J. M. (2000). *Real Science: What It Is, and What It Means*. Cambridge, UK: Cambridge University Press.
3. Krieger, N. (2011). *Epidemiology and the People's Health: Theory and Context*. New York: Oxford University Press.

4. Birn, A. E., Pillay, Y., & Holtz, T. H. (2017). *Textbook of Global Health*. 4th ed. New York: Oxford University Press.

5. Berkman, L. F., & Kawachi, I. (eds). (2000). *Social Epidemiology*. New York: Oxford University Press.

6. Berkman, L. F., Kawachi, I., & Glymour, M. (eds). (2014). *Social Epidemiology*. 2nd ed. New York: Oxford University Press.

7. Young, T. K. (1998). *Population Health: Concepts and Methods*. New York: Oxford University Press.

8. Young, T. K. (2014). *Population Health: Concepts and Methods*. 2nd ed. New York: Oxford University Press.

9. Oakes, J. M., & Kaufman, J. S. (eds). (2006). *Methods in Social Epidemiology*. San Francisco, CA: Jossey-Bass.

10. Oakes, J. M., & Kaufman, J. S. (eds). (2017). *Methods in Social Epidemiology*. 2nd ed. San Francisco, CA: Jossey-Bass.

11. O'Campo, P., & Dunn, J. R. (eds). (2002). *Rethinking Social Epidemiology: Towards a Science of Change*. Dordrecht: Springer.

12. Keyes, K. M., & Galena, S. (2016). *Population Health Sciences*. New York: Oxford University Press.

13. El-Sayed, A. M., & Galea, S. (eds). (2017). *Systems Science and Population Health*. New York: Oxford University Press.

14. Levy, B. S., & Patz, J. A. (eds). (2015). *Climate Change and Public Health*. New York: Oxford University Press.

15. Luber, G., & Lemey, J. (eds). (2015). *Global Climate Change and Human Health: From Science to Practice*. San Francisco, CA: Jossey-Bass.

16. Watts, N., Amman, M., Ayeb-Karlsson, S., Belesova, K., Bouley, T., . . . Boykoff, M. (2017). The Lancet countdown on health and climate change: From 25 years of inaction to a global transformation of public health. *Lancet*, Oct 30. pii: S01040–6736(17)32464–32469. [Epub ahead of print]. [Erratum in: *Lancet* Nov. 23, 2017.]

17. Holmes, D. E. (2017). *Big Data: A Very Short Introduction*. New York: Oxford University Press.

18. O'Neil, C. (2015). *Weapons of Math Destruction: How Big Data Increases Inequality and Threatens Democracy*. New York: Crown.

19. Frankel, F. (2009). *No Small Matter: Science on the Nanoscale*. Cambridge, MA: The Belknap Press of Harvard University Press.

20. Ge, Y., Li, S., Wang, S., & Moore, R. (eds). (2014). *Nanomedicine: Principles and Perspectives*. New York: Springer.

21. Pimental, D. A. V., Aymar, I. M., & Lawson, M. (Oxfam International). (2018). Reward work, not wealth: To end the inequality crisis, we must build an economy for ordinary working people, not the rich and powerful. *Oxfam Briefing Paper*, January. https://d1tn3vj7xz9fdh.cloudfront.net/s3fs-public/file_attachments/bp-reward-work-not-wealth-220118-en.pdf; accessed: February 4, 2018.

22. Piketty, T. (2014). *Capital in the Twenty-First Century*. Cambridge, MA: The Belknap Press of Harvard University Press.

23. Klein, N. (2017). *No Is Not Enough: Resisting Trump's Shock Politics and Winning the World We Need*. Chicago, IL: Haymarket Books.

24. Johnson, D., & Merians, V. (eds). (2017). *What We Do Now: Standing Up for Your Values in Trump's America*. Brooklyn, NY: Melville House.

25. President Donald Trump: The first 100 days. (2017). *Wall Street Journal*, May 1. https://www.wsj.com/livecoverage/donald-trumps-first-100-days; accessed: February 4, 2018.

26. Finnegan, M., & Barabak, M. (2018). "Shithole" and other racist things Trump has said—so far. *LA Times*, January 12. http://www.latimes.com/politics/la-na-trump-racism-remarks-20180111-htmlstory.html; accessed: February 4, 2018.

27. Krieger, N. (2017). The censorship of seven words by Trump's CDC could well cost American lives. Op-ed. *New York Daily News*, December 18. https://www.nydailynews.com/opinion/censorship-words-trump-cdc-cost-lives-article-1.3707447; accessed: February 4, 2018.

28. Beckfield, J. (2018). *Political Sociology and the People's Health*. New York: Oxford University Press.

ACKNOWLEDGMENTS

Nancy Krieger conceived this series of "Small Books with Big Ideas" about social epidemiology, invited me to contribute to it, and for the past ten years has been an intellectual inspiration, astounding collaborator, thoughtful mentor, and great friend. I am grateful to Nancy beyond expression. Sigrun Olafsdottir sparked my interest in the relevance of the welfare state for social inequalities in health with her own path-breaking work, and I am grateful to her not only for that intellectual inspiration, but also for her supportive friendship and crucial introduction to Icelandic society. Erin McDonnell, Dave Brady, Dalton Conley, George Davey Smith, and Nancy Krieger read the manuscript at a critical stage and offered supremely insightful and constructive feedback; I wish I could have adopted all their suggestions within the confines of this necessarily small book. I also thank Clare Bambra, Terje Eikemo, Tim Hiujts, and Claus Wendt, who have long inspired me with their cutting-edge work on welfare states, healthcare systems, and population health, and more recently welcomed me as a collaborator on the Health Inequalities in Welfare States (HiNEWS) project, funded by the New Opportunities for Research Funding Agency Cooperation in Europe (NORFACE) Welfare State Futures program. This book should be counted as a product of that project. Lisa Berkman leads a warm and engagingly interdisciplinary environment at the Harvard Center for Population and Development Studies, where I spent sabbatical time developing some of the ideas in this book. Parts of the book were also written at the Laboratoire Interdisciplinaire d'Evaluation des Politiques Publiques at Sciences-Po in Paris, Nuffield College in Oxford, and Café Las Flores in Managua; I thank my hosts for the friendly and stimulating hospitality. The Weatherhead Center for International Affairs at Harvard supported the sabbatical semester when I wrote most of the book. My doctoral advisor, Art Alderson, consistently and generously provided incisive, open-minded intellectual guidance as I pursued my doctorate at Indiana, where Jane McLeod, Bernice Pescosolido, and Eliza Pavalko sparked my interest in medical sociology. One way to read this book is as an imagined conversation between Indiana's medical sociologists and its political economy group. My former colleagues in the Department of Sociology at the University of Chicago, especially Lis Clemens, Andy Abbott, Linda Waite, and Andreas Glaeser, pushed my sociological imagination as an assistant professor in ways that deeply structure this book. My current colleagues in the Department of Sociology at Harvard University, especially Mary Waters, Mary Brinton, Sasha Killewald, Michele Lamont, Rob Sampson, Orlando Patterson, and Peter Marsden, have all challenged and shaped my thinking in ways that remain always unresolved and always generative. Ben Sosnaud had an enormous impact on my thinking about population health, through our research collaboration, and our co-teaching of "Death by Design" at Harvard. Genevieve

Butler assisted with the manuscript in many ways, including securing permissions from copyright holders and producing images. This book adapts selected material from published work (Beckfield et al., 2015; Beckfield & Bambra, 2016; Beckfield & Krieger, 2009; Beckfield, Olafsdottir, & Bakhtiari, 2013; Pinto & Beckfield, 2011; Sosnaud & Beckfield, 2017). I also thank audiences at Aarhus University, American University, Brown University, Columbia University, Harvard Medical School, McGill University, National Academy of Science, Northwestern University, Princeton University, Sciences-Po, Stanford University, Stockholm University, University of California–Los Angeles, University of California–Riverside, University of Chicago, University of Michigan, University of Pittsburgh, University of British Columbia, and Yale University, for their questions and comments as I presented earlier versions of some of these arguments—especially the political sociologist who encouraged (?) me by quipping that mine was "the least boring talk about health" he could remember. Most important of course is my family: thank you Jocelyn, Jackson, and Arabella for our wonderful lives together, including the rainy season in Nicaragua that taught us all so much about embodiment!

ABOUT THE AUTHOR

Jason Beckfield, PhD, is Professor and Chair of Sociology and Associate Director of the Center for Population and Development Studies at Harvard University. He conducts interdisciplinary research on how institutional arrangements—the "rules of the game" that organize power in social life—structure inequality, including the global distribution of population health. His work has been supported by the National Science Foundation, National Institutes of Health, Robert Wood Johnson Foundation, Harvard Medical School, and the American Sociological Association. He is also grateful to the taxpayers of the great states of Missouri and Indiana, who supported his training in the form of generous scholarships and fellowships.

INTRODUCTION

POLITICAL SOCIOLOGY AND SOCIAL EPIDEMIOLOGY

Depending on where she is born, an infant's chance of living to see her first birthday is as good as 99.8% in Iceland, or as bad as under 80% in parts of Afghanistan and Somalia. Depending on when he was born, 30 years ago an infant in the United States could expect to live almost as long as an Icelander, a Swede, or a Norwegian, but today he can expect to live a life about four years shorter, and that gap is growing.

These differences illustrate the big question: Why are health and illness distributed so unequally around the world? This central puzzle motivates this book. After decades of documenting profound, durable disparities in disease distribution across social categories of race, ethnicity, citizenship, class, status, gender, and sexuality, mostly in the United States and other rich democracies (Wilensky, 2002), scholars are now increasingly turning toward political causes and exposures for explanations (Beckfield & Krieger, 2009; Kunitz, 2015; Lundberg et al., 2015). For example, despite divergent foci and emphases, the ecosocial, fundamental-cause, and social-determinants theories of disease distribution all point toward politics and policies in explaining the social distribution of population health (Krieger, 2011; Link & Phelan, 1995; Marmot & Wilkinson, 2005). What concepts, theories, data, and measures do we find when we move in this new analytical direction? And what opportunities exist for political sociologists to show how the social organization of power is a matter of life and death?

The field of political sociology theorizes, conceptualizes, measures, and analyzes politics and policies at the macro- and mesoscopic levels of analysis (Clemens, 2016; Janoski, Alford, Hicks, & Schwartz, 2005; Leicht & Jenkins, 2011). Indeed, the aim of this book is to advance the field of research on health inequities and inequalities by developing the scholarly conversation between social epidemiology and political sociology. Specifically, political sociology offers to social epidemiology a macroscope: a new lens for understanding the production and distribution of population health. While I think research on health inequity and inequality has much to gain from engagement with political sociology, the gains also run in the opposite direction and offer political sociologists a rich array of theoretical and empirical tools for the advancement of their own agendas. Thus, while this book is written mainly for students and researchers interested in health inequality and inequity, it is also written for political sociologists interested in expanding their own toolkits by engaging fields that customarily travel outside the ambit of political sociology.

Political sociology investigates the social structure of power. More specifically, it investigates the social organization of power, where "social organization" means categorization, patterns of interaction, and formal structures that exist at the meso- and macro-levels of analysis, apart from the people who interact in such patterns and structures (Durkheim, 1938); and "power" means the capacity to achieve something against resistance (Weber, 2009). What makes these concepts fundamentally sociological is that they are, by definition, relational: "social organization" refers to relationships between and among people, and "power" only has meaning in the context of conflict and challenge between and among people. By this definition, many political scientists also "do" political sociology, and their contributions to the field tend to center on political contestation within formal institutions (more on the concept of "institution" later). While political sociology is central to the discipline of sociology, and a different book could be written about how sociology and social epidemiology could develop synthetic insights, I limit the scope of this book to political sociology because of its (a) emphasis on power relations, (b) explanations of social inequalities, (c) publicly available secondary data infrastructure, and (d) analytical position as upstream from and in some cases exogenous to the distribution of population health. For instance, consider a political-sociological definition of neoliberalism: neoliberalism can be conceptualized as an ideology of "market fundamentalism," where supply, demand, scarcity, and price are argued to best organize social relations and produce social welfare (Somers & Block, 2005).

Social epidemiology, as most readers of this book well know, investigates the distribution of health, disease, and death across societal categories of people (Berkman, Kawachi, & Glymour, 2014). The societal categories, which are societally defined in that they are neither social groups (people who know each other and interact regularly) nor biological groupings (despite the persistent efforts of eugenicists to establish otherwise), include genders, classes, races, ethnicities, sexualities, and nationalities, among other categories investigated by social epidemiologists. Social epidemiologists and social demographers also employ the concept of "birth cohort" to define categories for the analysis of disease distribution. Like political sociology, social epidemiology also crosses disciplines, not just into demography, but also public health, medicine, biology, psychology, and economics. Its focus on health, disease, and mortality as *explananda* render it a subfield of epidemiology (Oakes & Kaufman, 2006; Rothman, Greenland, & Lash, 2008). As Berkman et al. note, social epidemiology bridges over into neighboring fields: "Like environmental and nutritional epidemiology, social epidemiology must integrate phenomena at the margins of what is defined as its domain" (2014, p. 5).

I attempt with this book to develop the integration of concepts from social epidemiology and political sociology. For political sociology, an examination of health inequalities offers an array of new puzzles, which are theoretically engaging because they differ ontologically and etiologically from more familiar *explananda* like employment, wages, income, and wealth. Population health follows rich dynamics that allow for the investigation of how institutional change and institutional differences have distributional consequences. For social epidemiology, engagement with political sociology offers a fresh array of concepts, measures, and data that promise persuasive answers to questions about the "causes of the causes of" population health. As social epidemiologists increasingly look toward such causes in their investigation of the social determinants of health (Kunitz, 2015; Ratcliff, 2017), political sociology offers valuable concepts and tools.

Why have these fields tended to travel along separate paths, and why is now the time to consider new paths that might engage and benefit both fields? One reason is that much of social epidemiology is located in schools of public health or other organizations supported by their respective national governments (e.g., in the United States, the National Institutes of Health); in many such funding organizations, political topics carry stigma, and national research beats international or cross-national research in grant competitions, arguably because of the national priorities of the elected officials who allocate money to funding agencies. Since political sociology overtly concerns politics, and since much of political sociology is comparative, the opportunity structure for collaboration across these fields has been limited. Second, social epidemiology is a young, lively field that is still defining, expanding, and policing its boundaries. Third, some political sociologists, supported by universities in doing basic science, consider social epidemiology too applied, impure, or narrow to be interesting, while some social epidemiologists consider political sociology too esoteric, vague, or distal to be useful. Fourth, many political sociologists might not see how their agenda could be advanced by investigating disease distribution. Fifth, the dominance of the biomedical model of epidemiology tends to undermine both fields, because such research tends to use methods that hold constant the very meso- and macro-level exposures that political sociology problematizes. Sixth and finally, most social epidemiologists have not categorized the analysis of policy effects as within their domain of research questions, as Glymour notes:

Unfortunately, important gaps in knowledge exist about the long-term health effects of most major public policies shaping socioeconomic conditions. Furthermore, social epidemiologists have often regarded policy evaluation as tangential to their primary research, rather than as the central task for understanding the social determinants of health. (2014, p. 453)

In light of these potential reasons for the tendency of these two fields to develop separately, why is now the time for engagement? Part of the case rests on the growing influence of theoretical approaches to disease distribution that emphasize, in their respective and sometimes contradictory ways, political, economic, and social causes of bodily effects. First, ecosocial theory develops the concept of "embodiment"—the ongoing process whereby people incorporate characteristics of their environment at different levels of analysis simultaneously—to explain how historical changes in material conditions of life create health inequities (Krieger, 1994, 2011). These changes are fundamentally political, because they entail reorganizations of power, and distribution of power through institutional arrangements. Second, social determinants theory synthesizes work on nonmedical causes of health, viz. living conditions such as housing, work, position on the labor market, wealth, and neighborhoods, all of which are affected by politics and policies at the meso- and macro-scales (Marmot, 2005; Marmot & Wilkinson, 2005). Third, fundamental cause theory represents a radical epistemological shift in social epidemiology, away from the mechanisms that connect social causes to health effects, and toward the "causes of the causes," such as stratification itself (Link & Phelan, 1995). As the post-1980s shift in the field of social stratification to institutional analysis shows, the "rules of the game" set by social and economic policies strongly shape the quantity and quality of social inequality and stratification in a society, and thus should matter for embodiment (Alderson & Nielsen, 2002; Moller, Alderson, & Nielsen, 2009; Western, 1997, 2006).

In social epidemiology, relatively little empirical work has been done to connect such institutions to the distribution of population health (Beckfield & Krieger, 2009), though interest in policy and politics as social determinants is increasing (Osypuk, Joshi, Geronimo, & Acevedo-Garcia, 2014). In their review of this small but growing literature, Beckfield and Krieger (2009) identify the institutional arrangements that have been related to population health inequities in the rich democracies: (1) neoliberal restructuring of social policy, (2) the welfare state, and (3) political incorporation and, conversely, social exclusion, of subordinated groups. Political incorporation of minority groups and women is robustly associated with better health among those groups, suggesting a direct connection between political empowerment and health. In contrast to the broad consensus among studies of political incorporation, research on the welfare state is marked by controversy and debate, although on balance it does appear that there is at least a positive association between the generosity of the welfare state and population health (Beckfield & Bambra, 2016). Research in social epidemiology, especially in the United States, has tended to devote more attention to more "proximate" causes of health and illness, in part because in many datasets there is more variation in these proximate causes that makes them more useful to observational epidemiology. And so, a more expansive consideration of the distal/upstream determinants of population health can contribute much to the social epidemiology of social policy (Berkman et al., 2014). As Torres and Waldinger note, "politics and policies are often listed alongside the list of other fundamental causes, with little elaboration as to what these political forces might be and how they operate" (2015, p. 451). A core puzzle that such elaboration could address is how, why, and when cross-national differences vs. over-time institutional changes matter more for the distribution of population health.

In sociology, the "institutional turn" in the field of research on social stratification is still ongoing, and sociologists have investigated a relatively small set of institutions in this recent turn toward institutional explanation, in part because this work has also focused on economic goods such as wages and poverty, to the neglect of health, disease, and mortality (Brady, Blome, & Kleider, 2016; Grusky, 2001). The institutions that best explain cross-national differences and over-time change in income inequality and poverty, for example, include public welfare expenditure, minimum wage-setting, corporatist bargaining arrangements, childcare and family-leave policies, regulation of part-time and full-time employment, and public pensions (Alderson & Nielsen, 2002; Brady et al., 2016; Moller et al., 2009; Western, 2006). In the United States, given its roots in ethnic domination and settler-colonialism, slavery, and racism, racial institutions cause a large part of income inequality, poverty, and wealth inequality; such institutions include racial residential segregation (including of Native Americans), employment discrimination, and political exclusion, some forms of which are recently outlawed but still practiced, and remain embodied by American Indians and Alaska Natives and also African Americans (Krieger, Chen, Coull, Waterman, & Beckfield, 2013; Massey &

Denton, 1993; Pager, 2003; Pager, Western, & Bonikowski, 2009; Uggen & Manza, 2002).

The other part of the argument that now is the time for engagement between political sociology and social epidemiology rests on two critical intellectual developments that should engage both fields. The first is the turn toward epigenetics, or the study of molecular processes and properties such as methylation and histonal gene regulation (Goldberg, Allis, & Bernstein, 2007). It may sound strange to consider molecules in a book about politics and policies, but epigenetics raises political-sociological questions because the political environment could be conceptualized as part of the epigenome (Shostak & Beckfield, 2015), or at least as influences on biological embodiment. That is, politics and policies should shape gene expression. The second intellectual development that spurs engagement between political sociology and social epidemiology is the articulation of new and pressing puzzles about the global distribution of population health. One such puzzle is the finding of a growing mortality gap between the United States and other rich democracies: a recent National Academy of Sciences report calls for new research on political factors that may contribute to the gap (Woolf & Aron, 2013). Another such puzzle is the finding that Scandinavian welfare states, which have some of the more generous public welfare benefits in the world, also have some of the larger relative social inequities in health in the world: this "Nordic Paradox" is currently spurring large-scale research efforts (Eikemo, Balaj, Bambra, Beckfield, Huijts, & McNamara, 2017; Mackenbach, Kunst, Cavelaars, Groenhof, & Geurts, 1997). A third puzzle is the relationship between the distribution of health within a population and the average level of health of that population. Most generally, the finding of cross-national and historical variation in the patterning of health inequities represents arguably the foremost and broadest question for the current generation of social epidemiologists, and it is this question that motivates and frames this book.

1 | KEY CONCEPTS, MEASURES, AND DATA

In this chapter, I discuss several concepts, measures, and datasets that open new avenues for social epidemiologists to use political sociology to explain the distribution of population health. These concepts, measures, and datasets are summarized in Table 1.1. I also describe how epidemiological concepts can feed back into political sociology in a way that advances its agenda to understand the social organization of power. Three themes integrate the concerns of these still-disconnected fields: (1) the conceptualization of etiologic period, (2) the definition of population, and (3) the distinction between population averages vs. distributions within populations. Though these themes also engage epidemiology outside its social variant, social epidemiologists analyze etiology, population, and distribution through a specific focus on social inequality and social policy. Thus, this book focuses on social epidemiology, although many of the concepts span epidemiology generally.

When confronting the complexities of population health, my first inclination as a political sociologist was to assume that the distribution of health outcomes must depend primarily on the

Table 1.1 Concepts, Measures, and Data from Political Sociology

Concept	Definition	Measures	Data
Institution	Combination of schemas, resources, and practices that organize power	Comparative-historical analysis, content analysis, policy analysis	Secondary research using case-based evidence; Social Citizenship Indicators Program; Social Policy Indicators Network
Polity	Governance structure	Democracy, Autocracy, Federalism, Constitutionalism	Polity IV Project; Freedom House; Quality of Government Project
World Polity	Global governance structure	Ties to international organizations, diplomatic relations, colonial histories	Yearbook of International Organizations; CIA World Factbook; Correlates of War Project
Nation-State	Political authority with geographical boundaries and monopoly on the legitimate use of violence	State formation, national identification, national frames	United Nations Yearbook; Correlates of War Project; World Values Survey
Political Exclusion and Incorporation	Enforcement of the boundaries that restrict membership in a polity	Citizenship type, voting rights, representation	Inter-Parliamentary Union; Quality of Government Project

Gendered State	Loci of overlap between gender and the state; how policies and citizenship are gendered	Typologies: defamilization, general family support, dual-earner model, dual-carer model, market model	Comparative-historical research; e.g., Orloff (1993), Pettit and Hook (2004), Korpi (2000), Hacker (2017)
Racial Formation	Processes of constructing and institutionalizing races from socially defined categories	Variable definitions of racial categories, counts of racialized populations	National censuses
Political Economy	Loci of overlap between state and market	Typologies: coordinated vs. liberal market economies; liberal vs. conservative vs. social-democratic regimes; also measures of central bank independence	Comparative-historical research; e.g. Hall & Soskice (2001), Esping-Andersen (1990), Garriga (2016)
Welfare State	Complex of citizenship rights and social programs	Unemployment, family, pension, and health benefits; specific policies e.g. income replacement rates; policy expenditures as % of GDP or per capita	Comparative Welfare Entitlements Dataset; Comparative Welfare States Dataset; Comparative Political Datasets I–III; see also datasets listed previously in "Institution"

(continued)

Table 1.1 Continued

Concept	Definition	Measures	Data
Collective Bargaining	Negotiation of employment contracts between organized groups	Gross and net union membership, collective bargaining coverage, corporatist social pacts	Database on institutional characteristics of trade unions, wage setting, state intervention and social pacts, 1960–2010 (Visser 2011)
Policy Domains	Fields of organized interests and policymakers in a substantive area of policy	Organizational demography, network ties, resource flows, organized interest representation	Burstein (1991); Wendt (2009); Commonwealth Fund; WHO System of Health Accounts
Mobilization	Development of organized contestation in civil society	Membership in social organizations, social media content and ties	Earl and Kimport (2011); Lee (2016)
Public Opinion	Variably organized attitudes and beliefs among residents of a given polity	Feeling thermometer, approval/disapproval scores, ideological/partisan coherence	American National Election Surveys, World Values Surveys, General Social Survey, International Social Survey Program

innate or natural qualities of the object—the human body. This of course overlooks decades of work by social epidemiologists, who show how "life chances," in Weber's evocative phrase, are in fact socially structured. Such work presents opportunities for intellectual engagement between the fields because political sociology conceptualizes and measures how distributions are designed.

To visualize how structure and chance go together, Nancy Krieger introduced to social epidemiology an object and a metaphor that clarifies the general connections between political sociology and the distribution of population health: the quincunx. What is a quincunx? Its strange name and problematic provenance render it unfamiliar or even illegible to many social epidemiologists and political sociologists (Krieger, 2012). Sir Francis Galton invented the quincunx, named after a pattern of planting trees in formal gardens popular with Victorians, as a tool for illustrating how the arrangement of probabilities resulted in distributions. The tree pattern in question took the shape of the five dots on the fifth side of a six-sided die. The quincunx, or "Galton Board," placed many round pegs on a flat board, as shown in Figure 1.1. The insight is that if balls (or beans, as in the original) are dropped from the top of the board, and each round peg gives a 50/50 chance that the ball bounces to the left or to the right, then the result is a normal distribution. But, as the differently shaped quincunxes in the figure suggest, any distribution of the elements that pass through the figure can be obtained by changing the arrangement of the pegs, the bins, and the point at which the objects are dropped into the quincunx.

For example, Figure 1.1 shows how a quincunx can produce different distributions depending entirely upon the arrangement

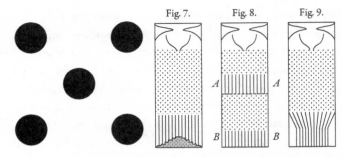

Figure 1.1 *The quincunx as physical representation of distribution generating process.*

of the pegs. In the left panel, we would obtain an approximately normal distribution of objects across the 13 bins at the lower part of the quincunx, with the largest concentration of objects in the middle bin, at the central tendency of the distribution. In the middle panel, objects falling into the bins at location A would also take on an approximately normal distribution, but an object falling into the leftmost bin at location A could appear in the rightmost bin at location B, depending upon the path it followed through the lower pegs. In the right panel, the objects dropped from the top of the quincunx would again fall to the bottom and take on an approximately normal distribution across the bins, but because the bins are narrower, the distribution would appear to be *leptokurtic* (or "peaked") relative to the distribution on the left.

Now imagine further modifications to the quincunx. We could generate a binomial distribution of objects simply by limiting the number of bins to two. Objects would still drop from the central funnel at the top, through the pegs, equally likely to fall to the right or to the left of each peg, but at the end of the process the objects could fall into just one of two bins. In this example, if we dropped thousands of objects into the binomial quincunx, we would expect about half to fall in the left bin, and half in the right bin, assuming the vertical wall separating the two bins was placed exactly in the middle of the space at the bottom of the quincunx. But say we wanted, not a ~50/50 distribution, but a ~75/25 distribution. We could obtain it by (a) shifting the starting point to the left or to the right, such that the objects had more opportunities, structurally, to end up in the left bin or the right bin; (b) changing the probabilities of falling left or right associated with each peg by modifying its shape, such as by replacing pins with uneven triangles; or (c) moving the wall separating the left bin from the right bin along the horizontal axis.

Using one or more of these modifications—starting point, path probability, or destination structure—we could also generate a skewed distribution. We could, for instance, design a quincunx that would generate a distribution of objects that would resemble the distribution of income across households residing in the United States, which has a long right tail with a few very high-income people, a median lower than the mean, and the bulk of households shifted toward the left, lower-earning side of the distribution. We could also design a quincunx that would distribute objects following the shape of the Canadian income distribution, the Australian income distribution, or the British income distribution, all of which have similar central tendencies to the U.S. distribution but exhibit much less skew.

The point is that distributions are not "natural" or "innate" and do not inhere exclusively in the objects being distributed; rather, distributions are created by processes that can be manipulated and modified. In the examples here, distributions are products of designs that are completely external to the objects distributed; the quincunx, or arrangement of probabilities, designs how many objects end up in which destinations. The quincunx shows how the fates of elements of a population can depend on design, rather than the attributes of the elements themselves.

Now imagine the distribution of adult mortality around the world. Let there be 20 bins, each of which captures a 5-percentage-point range of probability, such that the walls are placed at 0%, 5%, 10%, 15%, and so on through the last bin, which represents 95–100%. The mean probability, based on current rates of global adult mortality as measured by the number of people aged 15–60 who die per 1,000 people aged 15–60, is around 200 per 1,000, or about 20%. The current distribution of global adult mortality is right-skewed, with relatively fewer adults having a higher probability of mortality.

What is the design of this distribution? That is, what combination of starting points, path probabilities, and destination structures generates the global distribution of adult mortality? If we were to create a structure that would distribute the people of a population according to the distribution of global adult mortality, our first step might be to arrange multiple starting points, ordered from left to right, according to which country a person is born into, and that country's per capita income. This is a big part of the design, and requires making choices about how many countries and people there are, and how far apart the starting points are placed. The distribution of global income is not natural, but is designed by colonial exploitation, race and ethnic relations, unequal trade relations, currency regimes, and the fertility and migration dynamics of human populations. Our second step might be to design the path probabilities: what are the fateful turning points experienced by the people in our population? Two of the first would be gender and race, which are variably ascribed, according to different rules that vary by place and time. Race and gender make some paths more likely and other paths less likely, depending on how race and gender are institutionalized over the lifecourse. Social class—control over resources as often proxied by household wealth and income—would also create early turning points.

Institutional Context and Human Agency over the Lifecourse

Because people are more than physical elements of a physical system, the metaphor breaks down when we think about how and why people make choices in institutional contexts across the lifecourse. Although it is certainly true that randomness and simple luck play roles in the distribution of life chances (Jencks, 1972), people are not objects dropped through a quincunx. Indeed, one of the fundamental complexities of social science is that social structure and human agency are co-constitutive. But the quincunx does help in the visualization of how politics and policies structure life chances in spatially and historically varying ways, and we can even elaborate on the classical quincunx by allowing the elements to take on time-varying attributes that affect path probabilities in systematic ways. Take race, for instance. Race is a system of categorization that creates differential relations between people and their institutional contexts, so it could be incorporated into the quincunx as a variable magnetic field that would raise or lower the odds of different turning points for different elements of the population, depending upon physical properties of the elements themselves. Class and gender could work in the same way: class and gender are simultaneously attributes of people and institutional contexts, and only have the place- and time-varying effects they do when attributes combine in context. And because the elements of the quincunx (imagine alloy marbles that change over time in their metallic composition) can have only a finite arrangement of attributes at any point in time, the metaphor can stretch to allow for people to embody gender, race, and class simultaneously.

Currently, a forefront area for research is the interaction between socially structured people and consequential institutional contexts (Gage-Bouchard, 2017). How do people exercise human agency in relations with institutions? In terms of our metaphor, how do the elements bouncing around the quincunx make choices and ultimately restructure the quincunx for subsequent elements? Annette Lareau contributes important insights into how social class shapes how people interact with institutions, for instance in doctor–patient relationships: her middle-class study participants were more likely to approach powerful institutional agents (doctors, teachers, government officials) with a sense of entitlement, creating, through interaction, a qualitatively different relationship from that created by working-class and poor study participants (Lareau, 2011). Kristen Schilt identified how women and men experience workplaces differently by interviewing female-to-male transgendered people; here again, the relationship between institutional context and individual differed qualitatively depending upon the combination of attribute and institution (Schilt, 2006, 2010). Finally, Devah Pager showed how race shapes the experiences of individuals on the labor market: her audit studies revealed significant discrimination against blacks and Latinos in the Milwaukee and New York City labor markets (Pager, 2003; Pager & Quillian, 2005; Pager et al., 2009). It is not that the people in Lareau's, Schilt's, and Pager's studies had their fates determined by their attributes; the point is instead that the combination of agency and attribute depends probabilistically on how the properties of institutions and individuals combine.

The concept of heterogeneous treatment effects is useful in the analysis of how people live political institutions in ways that generate stratification over time. The core idea is that the same institutional factors—the same "rules of the game"—affect different people differently. To illustrate heterogeneous treatment effects, Yu Xie draws on survival analysis, where people vary both in propensity of receiving a treatment and in the effects of a treatment received (Xie, 2013). In the case of a stable population and a non-reversible cause where treatment cannot be undone, the highest-propensity units will enter into a treatment first, and the estimated treatment effects will depend on how the heterogeneous treatment effects are distributed across the treated and untreated populations. If the heterogeneous treatment effects are correlated, then estimates of causal effects are vulnerable to "composition bias," a form of selection bias. For instance, Brand and Xie show that treatment effects of higher education on earnings vary by the propensity to attend college, such that people least likely to attend college in two U.S. cohorts benefit the most when they do attend college (Brand & Xie, 2010; cf. Breen et al., 2015). The insight here is that institutional arrangements (e.g., the organization of higher education in the postwar United States), the metaphorical arrangement of the quincunx, can affect different people differently.

From the perspective of individual actors and individual-level action, theoretical developments from pragmatism can help in conceptualizing these qualitatively differing relationships between people and their political contexts. Neil Gross articulated a programmatic statement about how social mechanisms—processes that connect cause and effect—are better conceptualized from a pragmatist than from a rationalist conceptualization of action (Gross, 2009). While this book focuses on potential macroscopic political-sociological causes of disease distribution, it is important to note that such a focus does not entail the rationalist approach to action that often accompanies political-sociological analysis. In Gross's formulation, social mechanisms are chains of actors, their habits, the problems they encounter when their habits fail to cause the effects they expect, and the resolution that actors creatively make to solve their problems, which can include redefinition of the problems themselves.

For concreteness, consider how people confront social policy. In *Trapped in America's Safety Net*, political scientist Andrea Campbell shows how families exercise agency within the confines of the U.S. welfare state, where fragmentation and disconnection across policy domains can generate unanticipated consequences and deepen disadvantage (Campbell, 2014). The point is that social policy creates problems to solve, even as it offers solutions to problems. Thus, while I focus on macroscopic political structures and their potential roles in distributing health, such structures do not have automatic effects as in a physical system, but instead depend on human engagement, enactment, and construction through grounded problem-solving. This itself creates opportunities for observational and case-based political sociology, which sheds light on how micro-level (person-level), meso-level (organization- and neighborhood-level), and macro-level (national- and global-level) processes work together to cause inequality.

Biological concepts can help in identifying pathways whereby political contexts alter bodies at a molecular level (closer to what epidemiologists mean by micro-level). For instance, consider epigenetic epidemiology (Heijmans & Mill, 2012; Relton & Smith, 2010). If the Human Genome Project was Genetics 1.0, which promised to find "genes for" most if not all diseases and result in gene-specific medicine, Genetics 2.0 is revealing the molecular processes whereby the very composition and expression of the genome is altered by "the environment," which is loosely conceptualized in most epigenetic research (Shostak & Beckfield, 2015). For example, many studies rely on a residualist conceptualization of the environment, where "the environment" means everything that is "not genetic." While such research proceeds apace toward the development of drugs for "therapeutic targets," given the extensive resources devoted by governments, pharmaceutical companies, and other biomedical organizations that enable fast progress, there is already ample evidence about how the social environment gets "under the skin" (Ferraro & Shippee, 2009; Hatzenbuehler, 2009; Hertzman & Boyce, 2010; McDade, Williams, & Snodgrass, 2007; McEwen, 2012; Taylor, Repetti, & Seeman, 1997).

I argue that such evidence, combined with developments in social epidemiology, ecosocial theory, fundamental-causes theory, and the social-determinants approach, points to an urgent need for conceptual, methodological, and empirical work on the political-sociological environment that designs embodiment. Returning to the metaphor of the quincunx, the remainder of this book is about the political-sociological causes of epidemiological effects. The next section discusses the specific ways in which political arrangements structure the starting points, path probabilities, and destination structures that distribute population health, illness, and death.

Key Concepts in Political Sociology

I have selected the concepts from political sociology that are arguably the most promising for the explanation of embodiment in terms of the design of distributions. For comprehensive treatments of the field, I would recommend the excellent *What Is Political Sociology* (Clemens, 2016), *Handbook of Political Sociology* (Janoski et al., 2005), and *Handbook of Politics* (Leicht & Jenkins, 2011). Because political sociology is, like social epidemiology, a field that crosses disciplinary boundaries, current contributions can be found in leading sociology and political science journals, including the *American Journal of Sociology*, the *American Sociological Review*, the *American Journal of Political Science*, and the *American Political Science Review*. A few of the top international English-language journals are *World Politics, Comparative Political Studies*, and *European Sociological Review*.

Within US-based sociology, the subfields of political sociology and the sociology of health have matured without much dialogue. In terms of Andrew Abbott's colorful and apt metaphor for sociology as an archipelago with uneven interchange between some large islands and some small ones, political sociology and the sociology of health have grown into rather large, distant islands with few established shipping lanes for the exchange of ideas.

If this book succeeds in one of its aims, to engage political sociologists with puzzles and concepts from social epidemiology, the effective distance between these islands of sociology would begin to close. In service of that aim, in the following sections that focus on specific concepts from political sociology, I include unresolved questions from political sociology that might be advanced via engagement with concepts from social epidemiology. Each section, organized by political-sociological concept, concludes with a discussion of the measures and data available for the investigation of the political-sociological distribution of population health.

Fortunately, we live in a golden age of data availability for political sociology. Funding for scientific infrastructure, technological advancements, and strengthening transparency norms in science have all sparked a data explosion, such that the problem today is having far too much data rather than too little. Many of the publicly available datasets are reviewed by the Macro Data Guide. Unfortunately, though, the availability of data tilts much too far in the direction of quantitative data, which are much less useful for the qualitatively richer, process-oriented, historically informed research that often generates conceptual and theoretical innovation (Amenta, 2000; Go, 2013; Hall & Lamont, 2009; Krippner,

2011; Prasad, 2012). I think it is fair to say that the availability of secondary quantitative data tends to lag behind theoretical development, but reviewing such resources is still useful because even these are rarely if ever used by social epidemiologists (cf. Davey Smith et al., 1993), and many insights can be gained by using these resources to analyze the distribution of population health via the social organization of power.

In the text that follows, I discuss the key concepts summarized in Table 1.1, along with the datasets that provide quantitative measures of these concepts. I follow the order of the concepts as they appear in Table 1.1, and in the text I review several of the most-used publicly available datasets, emphasizing datasets that allow researchers to maximize institutional variation by comparing across polities and over time.

Institution

The concept "institution" occupies a central place in political sociology, and other subfields of sociology as well, including cultural sociology and economic sociology (Hall & Taylor, 1996; Powell & DiMaggio, 2012; Stinchcombe, 1997; Streeck & Thelen, 2005). Indeed, the concept is so central to and encompassing of so many intellectual projects that it requires careful definition at the outset. For political-sociological analysis, I define "institution" as a combination of schemas and resources that organize power, where "schema" means a symbolic system that constitutes categorization, and "resources" are material capabilities for the enactment and enforcement of schemas (Clemens & Cook, 1999). A central characteristic of an institution is its durability, as Brady et al. (2017, p. 124) note: "A strong institutionalism would claim that previously established rules and arrangements dominate over contemporary politics as those rules and arrangements 'lock in place' a level of egalitarianism."

Despite how abstract the definition of "institution" might sound to the epidemiologist's ear, there is nothing too exotic here. Consider the example of Active Labor Market Policy (ALMP), originally invented by Swedish Social Democrats as a way to promote market flexibility, social welfare, and full employment (Esping-Andersen & Korpi, 1986; Korpi & Palme, 1998). On the schema side of this institution is the idea, the model of social relations, that motivates the policy: people should be able to maintain a decent standard of living even when they are out of work because of inevitable but unpredictable market fluctuations. On the resources side of this institution are the public employees who carry out the policy, the public and private financing of the policy, and the organizations that structure the day-to-day work of the policy. The crucial object that combines schemas and resources in the case of ALMP is the law: laws enacted provide both the "rules of the game," the ideas that motivate and describe how social relations should work, and the resources to put policy into practice. Of course, "law on the books" never matches "law in action," so the conceptualization of schemas and resources as variables that can change orthogonally has utility for empirical scholars (Stryker, 2013).

To further clarify the concept of "institution," consider the institution of Jim Crow in the United States. Jim Crow was an institutional arrangement—a set of laws and their enforcement—whereby whites oppressed blacks with legal segregation in the organizations of everyday life (schools, restaurants, hospitals, and other places both public and private), and electoral processes that systematically excluded blacks from participation in formal politics, mostly but not exclusively in the Southern states. Jim Crow combined schemas (the idea of white racial superiority encoded in law) and resources (elections officials, police, administrators, and others who variably enacted the law).

How do the institutions of ALMP and Jim Crow organize power? The schemas categorize some people as legally and morally valid claimants to certain rights, and other people as legally and morally ineligible and unworthy as claimants to certain rights. The schemas also define the rights themselves: in the case of ALMP, the schemas define "labor," "employee," "employer," "unemployment," "economic activity," and "economic inactivity," and in the case of Jim Crow, the schemas define "black" (*viz.*, the one-drop rule) and "eligible voter" (*viz.*, payer of the poll tax and taker of the poll test). This organizes social relationships by constituting them: the relationships (employment, interaction, suppression, election) cannot exist independently of the schemas that enable them. At the same time, the resources are unevenly distributed across the actors and organizations involved in the interactions. For instance, workers had more power with ALMP because it gave them rights that were based in citizenship, not employment, and blacks had less power in Jim Crow because they were stripped of capacities for autonomous action. Since power and health go together, it makes sense that institutional arrangements like Jim Crow contribute to the distribution of premature mortality (Krieger et al., 2013; Riley, 2001).

Arguably, the central puzzles for institutional analysis are the explanation of institutional change and the identification of institutional effects (Streeck & Thelen, 2005). How and why do institutions—which are often by definition highly durable—change? And how and why do institutions—which are always macro-level and often emergent, constituted by but distinct from the actions of individuals—cause their effects? Social epidemiology concepts of etiologic period, population, and distribution can shed new light on these foundational questions. "Etiologic period" denotes the length of time required for the development of disease; causes of death, for instance, vary greatly in their etiologic periods, from accidents to the development of cardiovascular disease (Berkman et al., 2014). "Population" refers to a self-reproducing, bounded set of complex, animate individuals constituted by the causal relationships that create them, and the relational patterns that enmesh them (Krieger, 2012); in highlighting the co-constitutive quality of individual attributes and the causal processes that create populations, Krieger's definition allows for a careful conceptualization of attributes that only make sense in given populations, such as African-American in the contemporary United States. "Distribution" in epidemiology denotes the descriptive pattern that characterizes the frequency of attributes or states across the individuals in a given population (political sociologists use "distribution" to refer to the political-economic process of allocating goods, usually income, to people in states and markets).

The utility of social-epidemiological concepts for political sociology is illustrated by institutional change. Explanations of institutional change, which are core to the political-sociological project, often focus on political processes, including veto points, which tend to slow change, and layering, which can speed change by allowing for institutional transformation without abrupt replacement or disruptive invention. The concept of the etiologic period raises new questions about how institutional changes or political structures might vary systematically in the time required for their transformation or reproduction; for example, consider collective bargaining institutions such as labor unions and labor law, which may differ in their etiologic periods. Moreover, the concept of population itself may offer new explanations for institutional change and reproduction, if one considers the spatially and socially variable categorization that institutions do in defining and affecting populations. Finally, differentiating population averages from within-population distributions strengthens the analysis of institutional effects by broadening the range of *explananda* and opening new questions about divergent and potentially independent aggregate and distributional effects.

For example, consider two recent, major contributions to the political sociology of institutions. In *Re-Forming Capitalism*, Wolfgang Streeck argues that capitalism as an historical social order causes institutional change and reproduction through the actions of people and organizations in markets (Streeck, 2009). Specifically, his study of German capitalism since World War II reveals micro-level contestation over the very rules of political economy, the regulations that enable and constrain exchange in labor, products, and financial markets. Its primary contribution is to show, with detailed quantitative historical evidence on postwar capitalism in Germany, how the "German model" of coordinated capitalism was undone through the gradual and cumulative actions of employers, employees, and the state. Such processes can be conceptualized as endogenous institutional changes that take different forms: layering, conversion, drift, and exhaustion. Each form is defined and described by Streeck & Thelen (2005).

In *Varieties of Liberalization*, Kathleen Thelen argues that the undoing of the German model is one kind of liberalization, specifically a dualizing liberalization that also characterizes other conservative (conservative in the sense of maintaining status distinctions) welfare states in Continental Europe. Dualization involves the maintenance of a high level of protection and security for labor-market insiders, who are mostly unionized native-born men in the industrial sector, and the reduction of protection for less stable, lower-income, service-sector workers (Rueda, 2005). Thelen identifies two other types of liberalization as institutional change: deregulatory liberalization (as in the U.S.), and embedded "flexibilization" (as in Denmark). Each of the three ideal-types of liberalization happens through a distinct institutional dynamic: displacement causes deregulation, drift causes dualization, and conversion causes flexibilization. The central causal factor that sets political economies on these different tracks is coalition politics: disorganized labor and capital foster deregulation, strong but not encompassing organization of labor and capital in the manufacturing sector fosters dualization, and strong cross-sector labor organization and high-capacity states foster flexibilization.

What does social epidemiology have to add to these complementary explanations of institutional change in postwar capitalism? First, the concept of etiologic periods problematizes the length of time required by the body politic to translate coalitional cause into institutional effect. How do the institutional changes and their causes vary in the amount of time required to produce their effects, and how does this variation in the timing of institutional change shape the causes and effects of liberalization? Does the etiologic period, for instance, vary across national political economies; and if, so why? Second, what populations follow, reproduce, and change these institutions as they interact in markets? For example, the social-epidemiological concept of the population underscores that the populations of insiders and outsiders are constituted by their relations to dualist institutions (Rueda, 2005). The concept of population can also help to de-nationalize these theories of institutional change, by conceptualizing the set of people involved in institutional change by definitions other than the geographical. Third, the concept of distribution, while already well incorporated into the analysis of institutional effects on inequality (Western, 2006), can contribute to the political sociology of institutional change by problematizing the distribution of rule-makers and rule-takers itself as an important feature of the etiology of institutional change (Streeck, 2009).

While the foregoing suggests ways that social-epidemiological concepts can sharpen the political-sociological investigation of institutional change, the central focus of this book is on how political-sociological concepts can contribute to social epidemiology. To understand institutional change and the effects thereof on health inequalities, institutions must be measured. Measurement of institutions as defined here can be approached in at least three ways. First, a rights approach quantifies the law on the books: for instance, the Jim Crow status of a state could be measured as the presence or absence of laws restricting voting rights to whites, and active labor market institutions can be measured as the presence or absence of laws that give employers rights and employees obligations, and give employees citizenship rights to unemployment insurance, training, and other benefits. Second, a fiscal approach quantifies institutional arrangements by calculating the amount of money collected or spent by the government on a certain policy: for instance, the institutions of Jim Crow can be measured by poll-tax revenue, or public expenditures on the enforcement of voting restrictions, and ALMP can be measured by public spending on unemployment insurance and training. Third, observational and case-historical research describes and qualifies how people engage with institutional arrangements through socially structured enactment and resistance.

Data on institutional arrangements are available from a wide array of sources, some of which are identified hereafter. A good place to start in measuring any institutional arrangement is the relevant historical literature, which of course varies greatly by the institution considered, given that institutional arrangements are historically specific. Two general catalogs of institutional data used by political sociologists are the Macro Data Guide and the Quality of Government project (QOG, University of Gothenburg, Sweden, n.d.; The Macro Data Guide, n.d.).

Polity

The concept "polity" refers to a form of government, and while still quite broad is narrower in scope than "institution." It is a qualitative conceptualization of how rule is organized and conducted. Democracy, oligarchy, autocracy, monarchy, hegemony, empire, patriarchy, matriarchy, and racial oppression are all forms of rule. They differ in the distribution or concentration of power among the many or the few, the allocation of political rights, the role of law, particularism or universalism in recruitment to positions of power, the organization and representation of political interests, and mechanisms of enforcement. If a nation-state could be conceptualized as a body, the polity would be its skeleton.

Fundamental to measurement of a polity is the distinction between democracy and autocracy. As defined by political scientists Marshall and Jaggers in their highly influential Polity IV measurement project, democracy requires open and competitive political contestation (free elections), open recruitment to the executive (open elections), and constraints on the executive (constitutional, legislative, or judicial). Conceptualized as the opposite of democracy, autocracy requires suppressed political participation and contestation, closed recruitment to the executive (as in a hereditary monarchy), and a formally unconstrained executive. For example, consider the United States, which scores the maximum of 10 on Polity IV's democracy index, and the minimum of 0 on Polity IV's autocracy index, for nearly every year since 1871, except for dips in the democracy score to 8 in 1967–1973, and in 2016. Considering the *de facto* and *de jure* limits on political participation and executive recruitment in the U.S. electoral system, its score of a perfect 10 serves as a reminder that the Polity IV scores are formal, *de jure* measures of the organization of executive political authority only. For instance, the U.S. score does not reflect the fact that women did not win suffrage until 1920, or that American Indians were not granted citizenship until 1924. Nevertheless, these scores do vary systematically across polities: Russia scores 5 on democracy and 1 on autocracy, North Korea scores 0 on democracy and 10 on autocracy, and Venezuela under Chavez scored 0 on democracy and 4 on autocracy. Polity IV also measures two important demographic characteristics of polities: durability (time since establishment) and persistence (time since change in democracy or autocracy). If anything, macroscopic measurement of democracy suffers from an embarrassment of riches, as many scholars attempt to operationalize these complex concepts. A newer effort is the Varieties of Democracy project, which produces and disseminates hundreds of measures based on the ratings of country experts (Coppedge et al., 2016).

Polities organize power in different ways, and many democracies separate powers into branches of government. Drawing on Lijphart's classic work, the Comparative Welfare States Dataset includes typological indicators of federalism, presidential systems, bicameralism, plebiscite, and judicial review. The United States and Germany are cases of federalism, where the powers of the central government are limited by the strong roles of state governments in many policy domains, including regulations of labor markets such as minimum-wage laws. The United States further distributes power across the three branches of government, with a presidential executive branch that is not (ordinarily) elected by the representative bodies or appointed by the judiciary. This contrasts with the German case, where the Chancellor leads the executive branch and is elected by the lower house of representatives. Bicameralism also describes some polities, where there are two houses of representatives as in the United States and Germany, while unicameral polities have only one representative body, as in Finland and Sweden. Plebiscite is legislation through the direct voting of citizens, as in Switzerland, where, for instance, voters recently declined a guaranteed minimum income. U.S.-based readers will be familiar with judicial review, a characteristic of a polity wherein the judicial branch can review legislation adopted by the other branches under the Constitution. In political-sociological analysis, these indicators are often summed into a single measure of constitutional veto points, which tend to slow legislative change, including change in healthcare systems (Huber, Ragin, & Stephens, 1993; Immergut, 1990).

Electoral systems also vary across democratic polities, with proportional representation vs. first-past-the-post single-member districts differentiating most European polities from the United States, United Kingdom, and Canadian polities (Lijphart, 1995). In a proportional representation system, each district chooses representatives according to rules about what proportion of votes maps to what proportion of representatives from each party for the district, such that each district is represented by multiple members in legislative bodies, in proportion to the votes received by each party according to the (in most cases national) electoral rules. Conversely, single-member, first-past-the-post districts choose one representative each, specifically the one candidate who gains enough votes to be elected by the (again usually national) electoral rules. Work is just beginning to connect electoral systems to population health, and finds evidence that democracy is associated with longer life expectancy (Wigley & Akkoyunlu-Wigley, 2011).

In addition to the Polity IV project and the Comparative Welfare States Dataset, the Freedom House and Quality of Government projects are other often-used sources of data on polity type (Armstrong, 2011; Freedom House, n.d.; QOG, University of Gothenburg, Sweden, n.d.; Rothstein, 2011). Crucially, polities are historical formations, substantively inseparable from the populations across which they distribute power. The United States provides a particularly visible example, in the form of Jim Crow laws that described a coherent polity of racial oppression within the United States during the period between the end of Reconstruction after the Civil War of 1861–1865 and the 1964 and 1965 Civil Rights Acts. Jim Crow as a polity—a form of government that distributed power *a priori* to the electoral characteristics just described and also depended on federalism—had and continues to have a major effect on the distribution of health, illness, and death in the United States (Krieger et al., 2013; Kunitz, 2015). The same political distribution of population health holds for the apartheid polity in South Africa, and may grow in importance as polities debate the exclusion of migrants, refugees, and asylum-seekers, such that health care depends on "civic stratification" (Torres & Waldinger, 2015).

World Polity

Combining institutional analysis with the concept of a polity, sociological world polity theory describes and explains the development of governance at the international, transnational, and global levels of analysis (Meyer, Boli, Thomas, & Ramirez, 1997). The world polity is conceptualized as the network of states, societies, and international organizations that constitute a stateless form of governance that, despite its statelessness, caused many states and other organizations to adopt similar policies and formal structures, especially in the areas of education and market liberalization. While political sociologists examine the political-economic effects of the world polity (*viz.*, increased research and development activity, a general promotion of Western science, and investment in human capital through educational expansion), social epidemiologists explore the population-health effects of the world polity (Birn, 2009a, 2009b; Chorev, 2012; Harris, 2017; Shandra, Nobles, London, & Williamson, 2004).

The central contribution of world-polity scholarship has been to show how ideas, norms, and models spread through international organizations. The world polity is a stateless governance structure that is constituted by formally sovereign nation-state actors. Seeking legitimacy and legibility as actors in the world polity, states adopt formally and sometimes substantively similar structures and policies. Such adoptions of policies and structures are particularly visible when a new nation-state is established—e.g., a former colony declares independence, or a multi-ethnic state splits into new mono-ethnic states. The former resulted in a wave of new democratic polities established in the 1960s wave of democratization in Africa and Latin America; the latter resulted from the split of Yugoslavia into the republics of Bosnia-Herzegovina, Macedonia, Slovenia, and Croatia. Upon entering the world polity, these new nation-states established surprisingly similar formal structures, with similar parliaments, executives, ministries, and adoption of various international standards.

Two current debates in world polity scholarship surround decoupling and inequality. "Decoupling" is the separation between the formal declarations that nation-states make, often complying with international norms, and the actions that governments take to ignore or undercut such commitments (Meyer, 2010). To take one current example with major implications for global population health, the Paris Agreement on global warming and climate change signed in 2016 reflects formal commitments on the part of most of the world's governments to limit global warming through reductions in greenhouse gas emissions, but world-polity scholars would anticipate a great deal of decoupling between such statements and actual practice. The factors fostering tighter or looser coupling are just beginning to be understood (Clark, 2010; Hafner-Burton & Tsutsui, 2005; Schofer & Hironaka, 2005; Swiss, 2009). One argument is that such "soft law" mechanisms can actually generate more change through the social pressures of "naming and shaming," potentially reducing decoupling. Another argument is that social movements can use international agreements like Paris as a symbolic resource for political contestation. It may be that wealthier countries are more able to resist world-polity scripts, including in the domain of population health (Robinson, 2015).

Inequality in the world polity is also only just beginning to be understood. Formally, the world polity is equal at the level of norms and discourse: all nation-states are equally sovereign and participate equally in the stateless governance of the world polity. The world polity is universalist and integrative. But in actual practice, international organizations are highly unequal in the rates at which nation-states participate, in the influence nation-states have over international organizations, in their financing dependency on nation-states, and in their effects on nation-states (Beckfield, 2003, 2010). European dominance of the "world" polity is clear, building on not only a legacy of colonialism and empire, but also ongoing institutional economic policies (e.g., structural adjustment, whereby the International Monetary Fund [IMF] would offer funds to low-income countries only if they followed IMF prescriptions for austerity and privatization). There is, moreover, compelling ethnographic evidence that scholars in the Global North uneasily benefit from unequal power relations with African populations, after the "turn toward Africa" that placed embodied global inequalities at the center of Global North–dominated global health research (Crane, 2013).

This unequal world-political structure is made visible each time a public-health emergency arises: in the current case of the Zika virus, the contrast between the symbolic prominence of the World Health Organization (WHO) on one hand, and the WHO's financial and organizational dependency on nation-states on the other, is repeatedly exposed. The WHO's structural impotence toward transnational epidemics in effect nationalizes epidemics in a way that reproduces global inequities through embodiment. Moreover, to the extent that financial and organizational arrangements tightly couple the priorities of international organizations to the policies and actions of nation-states, the norms and standards promoted in the world polity have potential consequences for disease distribution through policies adopted by nation-states in compliance with international organizations (Ottersen et al., 2014). For instance, a striking fact about the development of the world polity since the 1970s is the combination of neoliberal economic orthodoxy, in the form of privatization, taxation, and financial liberalization policies, with liberal democracy, in the form of United Nations treaties on human rights, and the diffusion of democratic political institutions (Simmons, Dobbin, & Garrett, 2008).

How can concepts from social epidemiology advance the development of world polity theory? Consider again the concepts of etiologic period, population, and distribution. Most analyses of decoupling—differences between formal agreements and actual practices—downplay timing, other than the routine inclusion of "lagged effects" in quantitative models. The concept of etiologic period can help to develop new hypotheses about how national and international political processes produce decoupling. For instance, measures of formal policy agreements and actual practices could be modeled separately to identify how decoupling might result from cross-national differences in the etiologic periods of international agreements and national policy changes. The concept of population has entered world polity theory through demography and population ecology, and some of the earliest contributions used demographic concepts to understand the changing population of international organizations. Population-based analysis of the world polity could go much further, though; for instance, by investigating the population boundaries of international organizations, the categories of people created in and through international organizations, and the population directly employed by international organizations. Lastly, distributional concepts could drive world polity research even further than they already have; for example, by conceptualizing international organizations as distributive institutions (Viterna & Robertson, 2015).

The canonical data sources for world-political analysis are the *Yearbook of International Organizations*, and the Correlates of War project. The *Yearbook* contains rich information about thousands of international governmental and non-governmental organizations (NGOs), including their founding date, membership, location, official mission, organizational structure, and in some cases financing arrangements, governance, and specific projects. Such data allow for an analysis of the content and structure of the world polity, as an organizational field of cultural norms and stateless governance. For instance, one can use the data to measure the extent to which any nation-state—and states-in-formation and governments-in-exile—are integrated into the world polity. The Correlates of War data are more state-centric, and contain much more information about inter-state conflict and international relations. For instance, the data can be used to measure militarized international disputes (the political-science term for war), intergovernmental organizational networks, formal international relations through embassies and the like, and state military capacities. Unfortunately, neither dataset includes much information about what international organizations, governmental or intergovernmental, actually do. Thus, a forefront area for world-polity research as it relates to global health distribution is observational research and case-historical work on how international organizations contribute to global disease distribution via their effects on the policies of nation-states, and their state-like activities in the area of global health provision (Chorev, 2012; Krause, 2014; Star, 1999; Timmermans & Epstein, 2010). Such work could draw on guides to the systematic integration of quantitative and qualitative evidence (Lieberman, 2005; Small, 2011).

Nation-State

The nation-state is a central object of scholarship for most political sociologists, and arguably the primary kind of polity studied, although by world-historical standards it is a relatively recent institutional invention that superseded city-states, empires, and theocracies (Tilly, 1990). The nation, or the "imagined community" (Anderson, 2006), often developed alongside and from the political projects that formed states, through many processes such as the development of rail systems and public schooling (Dobbin, 1994; Meyer, Tyack, Nagel, & Gordon, 1979). However, the state is often analyzed separately from the nation, since the territorial and social scope of nation and state overlap imperfectly. The classical definition of "state" is the organization with a monopoly on the legitimate use of violence, in modern states through the police and military. Political sociologists investigate the state as *explanandum* (how do states form and why do they change?) and *explanan* (how does state capacity shape democracy, and how do agents of the state pursue their own interests?).

Cross-national and historically comparative research from political sociology and political science has developed an array of conceptual approaches to understanding cross-national differences in institutional arrangements, including nation-states (Kenworthy, 2004; Pontusson, 2005). Before describing concepts for understanding the nation-state, I note that the bounded-ness of the nation-state is, of course, itself a thorny problem. Some of the most innovative ongoing research problematizes the very national boundaries of institutions, thereby surpassing the "methodological nationalism" that characterizes much research from the social and population sciences (Bonikowski, 2010; Wimmer & Glick Schiller, 2002). Such work is of course directly related to theoretical issues in epidemiology surrounding the very definition of "population" (Krieger, 2011).

A forefront area of research is supra-, sub-, and non-national populations and policy (Beckfield, 2013; Lynch, 2008). This is because geographic boundaries are central to the concept of a nation-state: they influence who is subject to what institutional arrangements, and when (D. Hacker, 2017). National boundaries are historically contingent, making long-term over-time comparisons of nation-states problematic without paying attention to changing geography. For example, decolonization in Africa and Latin America created new national boundaries in the 1960s, and the fall of the Soviet Union created several new nation-states with new national boundaries in the 1990s. In the United States, 50,000 Mexicans became U.S. citizens after the Mexican-American War resulted in the United States gaining territory that now constitutes the states of Texas, Arizona, New Mexico, California, and parts of other states (Massey, 2009). Thus, current populations in these and other places have experienced widely diverging institutional settings over the lifecourse and across generations, as a result of combined migration, nationaliza-tion, and de-nationalization. Citizenship regimes also vary widely across nation-states and within nation-states over time, creating a complex political ecology of citizenship that could grow more consequential to the distribution of population health in a time of global climate change. For example, in Canada, the province of Quebec has developed a distinctive citizenship regime that connects states, markets, and communities in a way that is distinct from the Canadian citizenship regime; *viz.*, the Quebec citizen-ship regime is a discourse wherein states and markets take the role of supporting a distinct Francophone community (Jenson, 1997). Thus, the nation-state must be understood as an historical forma-tion that entails variable territory, authority, and rights, in Sassen's evocative phrase (Sassen, 2006). There is evidence from recent U.S.-based research that such political-institutional variation, ex-perienced as civic stratification by individuals with varying legal rights, shapes health care (Torres & Waldinger, 2015).

In relatively more settled times, absent boundary flux and war, state structures and processes profoundly affect social policies (Skocpol & Amenta, 1986). The key insight of the historical-institutionalist approach to nation-states is that political contestation inside and outside formal electoral politics both causes and is caused by social policy. That is, historical sociology reveals the causes and consequences of political events, processes, transformations, and feedbacks (Clemens, 2007). The social-epidemiological concepts of etiologic period and population resonate with the historical-institutionalist tradition in political sociology, which theorizes how social policies can create their own constituencies, populations who protect the policies from change, over timeframes that vary by policy domain and state structure. For example, "centralization," "bureaucratization," and "electoral synchronization" all describe state structures and processes that can matter for the distribution of power and thus the distribution of population health. Currently, in many rich democracies, relevant policy feedbacks go from policies on trade, migration, and welfare cutbacks, to right-wing populist movements that aim to protect the nation-state through the politics of identity and security (Berezin, 2002, 2009).

Incorporation and Exclusion

Incorporation and exclusion characterize processes that position socially relevant categories of people vis-à-vis a polity. Political incorporation is the process of extending political rights (e.g., citizenship, voting, claims-making) to marginalized groups defined by race, ethnicity, nationality, language, gender, or sexuality. For example, the 1965 Voting Rights Act legally ended the

Jim Crow system of electoral exclusion of African Americans. The end of legal apartheid in South Africa extended political rights to black South Africans. Women's suffrage movements around the world advanced political incorporation in extending voting rights to women. When the U.S. Supreme Court legalized gay marriage in the United States in the *Obergefell* case, it legalized political incorporation of lesbians and gays. Currently, these and other kinds of political contestation over rights are ongoing around the world, including heated debates over migrant rights in Europe.

Exclusion is the reverse of incorporation: it is a social process whereby socially relevant categories of people are removed from full political membership. The institutionalization of Jim Crow was an example of an exclusion movement, as it expressly raised barriers to the exercise of voting rights and other rights of political participation. Currently, many polities around the world exclude migrant minorities from full membership; examples of such exclusionary institutions are *hukou* legal status of rural-to-urban migrants in China, birthright citizenship in the United States, and asylum quotas in the European Union (Bauböck & Guiraudon, 2009; Glenn, 2011; C. Han & Whyte, 2009; Whyte, 2005, 2010). Felon disenfranchisement in the United States is another mechanism of political exclusion, one that is formally grounded in legal status but informally and disproportionately affects African Americans given racist policing and sentencing practices (Uggen & Manza, 2002; Western, 2006). Such exclusionary arrangements remove political rights from people who are otherwise legitimate claimants to such rights, or prevent potential claimants from obtaining means of political participation.

Incorporation and exclusion—as macroscopic political exposures with heterogeneous effects depending on socially inscribed individual characteristics—can be measured as the laws and practices of the state. For example, citizenship regimes, residential segregation, miscegenation laws, legal processes in racial formation such as the legal designation of different categories of people, language requirements and poll taxes for political participation, and government agencies charged with the incorporation of disadvantaged groups all entail incorporation and exclusion (Gerstle & Mollenkopf, 2001; Hochschild & Mollenkopf, 2009). Such "boundary institutions" reinforce group distinctions and undermine collective efforts to address population health problems (Gauri & Lieberman, 2006). While most of the research has focused on the incorporation/exclusion of racial minorities and migrants, there is also a literature on gender mainstreaming, an influential set of approaches for the political incorporation of women and gender, for example through supranational non-discrimination regulation in the European Union (Walby, 2005).

Data on incorporation and exclusion can be found in a variety of sources, including the Migrant Integration Policy Index (MIPEX), and the International Migration Policy And Law Analysis (IMPALA) Database (IMPALA Database, n.d.; Migrant Integration Policy Index/MIPEX 2015, n.d.). In the MIPEX, indicators include regulations regarding family reunification, acquiring legal permanent residence, voting rights, non-discrimination laws, and access to national systems of health care and education in the host country. MIPEX covers the member states of the European Union, plus other rich democracies that are traditional migrant-destination countries. Time coverage is

2004–2014. The IMPALA database is newer and still in development, and includes most of the same countries in the MIPEX data: Australia, Austria, Belgium, Canada, Czech Republic, Denmark, Finland, France, Germany, Greece, Hungary, Iceland, Ireland, Italy, Japan, Luxembourg, the Netherlands, New Zealand, Norway, Portugal, Slovakia, Spain, Sweden, Switzerland, the United Kingdom, and the United States. While MIPEX focuses on *de facto* and *de jure* indicators of migrant incorporation in host countries, IMPALA focuses on the legal regulations of immigration itself, with detailed data on the specific barriers to immigration via different tracks (Beine et al., 2016).

Social media, social network, and topic modeling of online data are newer ways to measure macroscopic social incorporation and exclusion. For example, data from Twitter, Facebook, and online dating sites have been used to proxy structure and change in incorporation and exclusion (Bail, 2014; Lewis, 2013, 2015). Likewise, social networks—for instance, intermarriage, a "strong tie" in a formal network-analytic sense—can indicate changing racial boundaries in intimate exclusion and inclusion (Lee & Bean, 2004, 2010). Separately, machine-learning algorithms for the estimation of topic models can be used to identify patterns in text data that may correspond to social incorporation and exclusion (Ramage, Dumais, & Liebling, 2010); an example of such patterning is contestation between #BLM (Black Lives Matter) and #TCOT (Top Conservatives on Twitter) in the United States following police shootings of unarmed African American men (Ray, Brown, Fraistat, & Summers, 2017).

Social-epidemiological concepts can advance the social science of incorporation and exclusion by providing systematic ways of thinking about and measuring how, when, and for whom such processes matter. For example, the concept of etiologic period helps to define the social groups most relevant to an examination of institutional effects in this domain, since incorporation and exclusion play out over different time scales for different groups depending on the precise mechanism in question. Also, the epidemiological conceptualization of population raises new questions about how exclusion and incorporation can create populations (similar to the ways in which racial formation projects rest on political and legal foundations; see later discussion herein). Finally, the concept of disease distribution can be applied to incorporation and exclusion to generate new questions, such as about the relationship between citizen voting rights, which would have the most influence on a weighted average of political rights, and non-citizen voting rights, which would contribute more information on the amount of political inequality in a polity under various forms of representation (Mansbridge, 2003).

Gendered State

The concept of "gendered state" refers to the ways in which states variably reflect, encode, and reproduce gender relations (Bird & Rieker, 2008; Orloff, 1993; Pettit & Hook, 2009; Seidman, 1999). Bird and Rieker synthesized decades of research on gender inequalities in mortality and morbidity, under their constrained-choices framework that problematizes the variable ways in which the social policy context makes different choices available to different women and men in different settings. In political sociology, these contexts are conceptualized under the rubric of "the gendered state," which refers to the political effects of gender as a system of categorical inequality that ascribes normative roles on the basis of sex. That is, gender as a framework shapes what states are and what they do. For instance, scholars have traced the effects of center-right governments in Europe, which tend to hold traditional or market-egalitarian gender ideologies, on the extension of parental leave benefits that are available only to women, and provide limited and means-tested benefits. These have the effect of reinforcing traditional gender ideologies that assign gender to carework (Morgan & Zippel, 2003). The gender of the state has deep historical roots, as revealed in Kimberly Morgan's *Working Mothers and the Welfare State*, which reveals organized religion in now-secular states as an important cause of divergent gendered political economies (Morgan, 2006).

Even when parental leaves are designed in a more generous and gender-equitable manner, as in Sweden where men are incentivized to take family leave and where take-up rates are higher among men, the gendered state can reinforce tradeoffs between the incorporation of women into the paid labor market on one hand, and occupational sex segregation and other measures of gender inequality in the paid labor market on the other. In *Gendered Tradeoffs*, Pettit and Hook use individual-level and social-policy data from several rich democracies to demonstrate that there is substantial heterogeneity across welfare states in the inclusion of women in the paid labor force, and that variation to a large extent coincides with other measures of gender inequality, including the gender wage gap, and gender differences in the accumulation of human capital (Pettit & Hook, 2009).

Currently, an important move in the literature on gendered states is the consideration of the intersectional gendering of states.

That is, the policies that reflect and affect the gender of states are also variably classed and raced, such that non-citizen women face variable problems and resources depending upon their social class, in ways that may affect the social stratification of health (Gkiouleka, Huijts, Beckfield, & Bambra, 2018). Simultaneous attention to gender and class, for instance, reveals how, depending upon the specific design of parental and family care leave policies, women with vs. without tertiary educational attainment are advantaged and disadvantaged (Korpi, Ferrarini, & Englund, 2013; Morgan & Zippel, 2003). For example, the length of family leave affects the nature of the Pettit-Hook gendered tradeoff, as longer leaves are associated with labor-market disadvantages for women, such that medium-term leaves (6–12 months) appear to be optimal in several labor-market outcomes (Misra, Budig, & Boeckmann, 2011). Citizenship intersects with class and gender as well, such as in the provision of essential carework by migrant women in many rich democracies.

Some of the best research on gendered states appears in the leading sociology and political science journals, listed before, as well as in journals such as *Gender and Society* and *Social Politics*. The journal *Community, Work and Family* also published a helpful special issue in 2011 on the topic of "anticipated and unanticipated consequences of work-family policy: insights from international comparative analyses" that should inspire future work in this area. The central resource for comparative cross-national work on gendered states in rich democracies is the Luxembourg Income Study, which provides researchers with harmonized and in many cases standardized individual-level data that inform the development of gendered-state typologies. Thus, the results from these studies could be used as measures of the gendered state at the macro level, for the political-sociological study of health distribution. Indicators of gendered social policy, such as detailed policy indicators in the domains of family and child care, where women tend to bear the greater burden but variably so across societies, are available in many of the welfare-state databases reviewed here. The Social Policy Indicators (SPIN) database is notable for its inclusion of detailed data in this domain (accessible at http://www.sofi.su.se/spin/). Other secondary data, even children's books, also provide windows into gendered states, as inequity in female representation in children's books reached its height between waves of feminist mobilization in the 20th century United States (McCabe, Fairchild, Grauerholz, Pescosolido, & Tope, 2011). While many measures of gendered states have not been connected to population health, Miller uses the timing of state laws guaranteeing women's suffrage in the United States to identify the roles of gendered policy preferences in supporting public health expenditure and child survival (Miller, 2008).

Racial Formation

"Racial formation" refers to the production of race as a social category through political means, including the definition of who qualifies for citizenship and who can access citizenship rights, including voting and public goods. Following the racial formation approach to the political sociological analysis of race, race appears as a political variable rather than a biological constant. That is, people are only categorized into races via political projects that ascribe phenotypical characteristics as racial; these political projects include regular population censuses legalized, organized, executed, and interpreted by states and the agents of states. Here the connections between the population and the political are clear, as Rodriguez-Muniz shows for the case of the "Hispanic population" in the United States (Rodríguez-Muñiz, 2016). Another prominent case of visibly political population-counting is France, where the official identification or enumeration of racial groups is forbidden by the centralized French state.

While much of the existing work on racial formation uses comparative-historical methods to reveal the political processes that construct racial categories and racialize populations, text analysis, social media data, and social network analysis are newer ways of measuring macroscopic patterns of racial formation, and even race relations. For instance, the U.S. Census Bureau recently considered adding a new race/ethnicity category to its 2020 decennial enumeration of the U.S. population: Middle Eastern or North African. The Bureau ultimately rejected this idea, but the contestation over it reveals how states variably institutionalize social categories. In this way, census reports can be analyzed by computational techniques for the analysis of text data, to reveal the construction of and change in racial and ethnic categories over time. Convenient for research, modern states tend to produce publicly available reports, white papers, legal statutes, and regulatory guidelines that provide rich veins for the identification of institutionalization via the state. That is, administrative residue can reveal how states develop and organize racial categories.

Currently, social media offer new opportunities for the measurement of race relations, as exemplified by Rashawn Ray's study of online groups after the shooting of Michael Brown in Ferguson, Missouri, wherein the authors found that online social organizing faithfully tracked on-the-ground mobilization (Ray et al., 2017). At a macroscopic level, several measures of ethnolinguistic fractionalization have been developed as comparative-historical quantitative indicators of race relations (Alesina, Devleeschauwer, Easterly, Kurlat, & Wacziarg, 2003; Fearon, 2003; Posner, 2004). For political sociologists, engaging population health would help to sharpen the ongoing debate about the consequences of ethnolinguistic diversity for public goods (Brady & Finnigan, 2014; E. M. McDonnell, 2016).

Political Economy

In selecting cases for the comparative analysis of population health, typologies of political economy can be helpful. For instance, the "Varieties of Capitalism" (or VoC) institutionalist tradition focuses on the role of employers and employees in welfare politics and policy within the context of international market competition (Hall & Soskice, 2001). The key taxonomic distinction is between "coordinated market economies" like Germany and Sweden and "liberal market economies" like the United States and the United Kingdom. The axis of differentiation that creates varieties of capitalism, instead of just capitalism, is the problem of coordination in actually existing markets. Market exchange—of goods, labor, and capital—requires the production and consumption of information, the regulation of contracts, the alignment of conflicting interests, and the settlement of contestation between incumbents and challengers. In coordinated market economies (CMEs), conflicts are resolved—or at least guided—via coordination among organized market actors, including peak business associations, peak labor associations, and the state. In liberal market economies (LMEs), coordination problems are left to less-regulated market exchange, where the state, for instance, enforces but does not negotiate contracts. CMEs and LMEs are different ways of organizing the distribution of power in markets, in that individuals and organizations with monopsony or monopoly positions can exploit their closure more fully in LMEs, resulting in higher levels of market inequality caused by the production of economic rents. In CMEs, organizations and states diffuse power, in particular empowering skilled labor to invest in specific skills with the security of social protection from unemployment caused by market fluctuations. CMEs tend to produce less wage inequality but also usually more occupational gender segregation via gendered public employment and the reinforcement of dualist insider–outsider dynamics (Pettit & Hook, 2009; Rueda, 2005; Streeck, 2009).

Varieties-of-capitalism research follows in the strong comparative-historical typological tradition in political economy. An earlier, influential typology of political economy developed from Gøsta Esping-Andersen's research on welfare regimes (described in greater detail below in the "welfare states" section). He identified three regimes—or systems of order at the junction of state and market— encompassing European political economies that developed after World War II. For Esping-Andersen, the key axis of differentiation between regimes is the extent to which labor is decommodified. Liberal regimes (the United States, United Kingdom, Canada, Australia, New Zealand) decommodify little, and people depend on wage labor to maintain socially acceptable standards of living. Conservative regimes (Austria, Belgium, France, Germany, the Netherlands) decommodify substantially, but in ways that reinforce status distinctions between family types and occupations. Social democratic regimes decommodify most, through universal benefit systems that reduce status distinctions. Table 1.2 summarizes the VoC and regime typologies. Note that both exclude guaranteed minimum income (sometimes called basic-income) policies, which have been and continue to be the subject of policy experiments (Atkinson, 1996; Forget, 2011).

An organizing variable of political economy that cuts across regimes and varieties of capitalism is central bank independence, or the relative autonomy of appointed officials who set monetary policies that determine the interest rates charged to banks by the central government, as well as the quantity of national currency. This independence has both a *de jure* component, which is measured by coding the laws establishing and modifying the rights of central bankers, and a *de facto* component, with is measured by observing actual interaction between the government and the central bank. In the United States, the central bank is the Federal Reserve System, which is controlled by the Board of Governors, who are appointed by the President and confirmed to single 14-year terms by the Senate. A key objective of many central banks is price stability, a situation where the money supply is fairly stable and neither deflation (decreasing prices) nor inflation (increasing prices) predominates. Central bank independence matters for the organization and distribution of power because, first, it is a primary prescription of neoliberalism for poor countries; and second, inflation is not politically neutral but instead favors wage-earners over capital-holders (Hung & Thompson, 2016). Central bank independence is often a condition of international loans from wealthy countries to poor ones. In macroeconomic terms, there

Table 1.2 **Political Economy Typologies: Varieties of Capitalism, and Welfare Regimes**

Typology	Differentiation	Types	Cases
Varieties of Capitalism	Market vs. state as primary mechanism of coordination among organizations	Liberal Market Economies (LME)	U.S., U.K., Canada, Australia, New Zealand
		Coordinated Market Economies (CME)	Germany, France, Netherlands, Japan, Austria, Belgium, Denmark, Sweden, Finland, Norway, Iceland
Welfare Regimes	Decommodification of labor	Liberal	U.S., U.K., Canada, Australia, New Zealand
		Conservative	Germany, France, Netherlands, Japan, Austria, Belgium
		Social Democratic	Denmark, Sweden, Finland, Norway, Iceland

is also often a tradeoff between employment and inflation, such that a deflationary or zero-inflation economy will have more unemployment, *ceteris paribus*, than a moderate-inflation economy.

Data on central bank independence are available from several sources, most recently a dataset published by Ana Carolina Garriga (Garriga, 2016). The Garriga data are global in scope, with annual data on a maximum of 182 countries over the 1970–2012 period, when central bank independence was a contested intervention promoted by reformers of various political stripes. Importantly, these data concern *de jure* independence, which can differ substantially from independence and political dependence in practice, as a case of the frequent divergence of "law on the books" from "law in practice." In contrast to other data on *de jure* central bank independence, the Garriga data include cross-nationally comparable indicators both of measures that enhance, as well as measures that constrain, bank independence. For instance, long or unlimited terms of office for the chief executive of the central bank are usually seen as a key aspect of bank independence. The goals of the central bank, and control over setting those goals in the areas of inflation and exchange rates, also affect central bank independence and can be compared across political economies.

Economic output is another commonly used measure of political economy, though many have noted its limitations (Anand, Segal, & Stiglitz, 2010). The most common measure of economic output, sometimes referred to as "economic development," is gross product, or the total value of all goods and services produced in a geographically defined economy. In the United States, data are available for the gross domestic product (GDP) from the Bureau of

Economic Analysis (BEA), by county, state, and industry classification. The BEA also publishes price-level comparisons, which are useful for comparing market conditions across states and locating people within variable markets (U.S. Department of Commerce, n.d.). For instance, such fine-grained comparisons are important in identifying the causal effects of recessions on health, because many of the theoretical mechanisms that may connect recessions to mortality concern local employment prospects in local labor markets (Noelke & Beckfield, 2014). Figure 1.2 depicts cross-state variation in GDP per capita, using 2016 data from the BEA, and makes clear the substantial within-nation variation in economic conditions in the United States, where the highest-GDP state (Massachusetts, $65,545) has nearly twice the GDP of the lowest-GDP state (Mississippi, $38,881). Of course, more granular areal comparison would reveal even starker economic inequality (e.g., the District of Columbia is an outlier on the map, with a per capita GDP of over $160,472).

There are many sources of international data on economic output. For cross-national comparative research, the canonical source is the Penn World Table (PWT), which provides estimates of macroeconomic attributes that are based on the principle of purchasing power parity (PPP). Rather than the traditional approach of assuming that all goods and services produced in one national economy are available in all other national economies, and then calculating price conversions based on currency exchange rates, the PWT project simulates a common "basket of goods" that is broadly available, and then uses those price comparisons to convert national economic product data denominated in national currency units into a common international currency. Perhaps the

Per capita real GDP by state (chained 2009 dollars) – All industry total, 2016

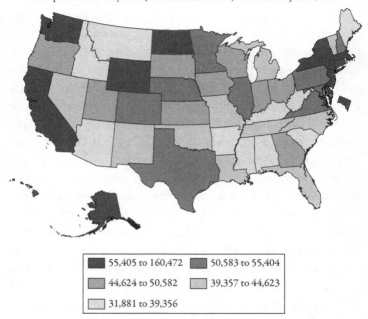

■	55,405 to 160,472	■	50,583 to 55,404
■	44,624 to 50,582	□	39,357 to 44,623
□	31,881 to 39,356		

Figure 1.2 *The distribution of economic resources across U.S. states, 2016.*

Source: https:www.bea.gov/itable

most commonly used measures in the PWT data are real GDP and real GDP per capita, where "real" means PPP-adjusted and inflation-adjusted. Another commonly used measure from the PWT is government consumption as a percentage of real GDP, which has been used as a rough proxy for state size and capacity. Figure 1.3 shows the distribution of GDP per capita around the

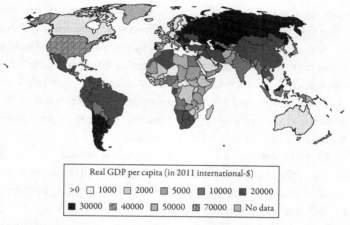

Figure 1.3 *The international distribution of price- and inflation-adjusted GDP per capita in 2014.*

Source: Penn World Table.

world, using data from the PWT. Again the economic inequality is striking, with the richest countries at approximately 70 times the GDP per capita of the poorest countries.

Welfare State

The welfare state is conceptualized as a complex of citizenship rights that provide social goods to people on the basis of membership in a polity (Marshall, 1963). Such "social rights of citizenship" are usually contrasted to property rights in markets: the welfare state may provide money to an unemployed citizen, and this "social wage" differs from the "market wage" an employee may receive. Of course, as the preceding discussion of political economy argues, the analytical distinction between state and market and public and private, blurs in practice, as many welfare states require employers to provide certain rights and benefits to employees (J. S. Hacker, 2002). Nevertheless, the conceptual and analytical distinction is an important one, because welfare states combine citizenship rights and property rights in systematically varying ways across nations and over time.

One influential political-sociological approach to understanding this variation between and within welfare states is the "welfare regime" framework developed by Gøsta Esping-Anderson in 1990, which posits the existence of "three worlds of welfare capitalism": liberal, social democratic, and conservative (Esping-Andersen, 1990). Welfare states are categorized into one of these three regimes according to the extent to which they decommodify labor by making it possible to maintain a socially acceptable standard of living without reliance on the market. Liberal (free-market) welfare states provide only minimal, and often means-tested, benefits; conservative welfare states provide generous benefits but only to certain categories of people in a way that tends to reproduce status distinctions; social democratic welfare states provide generous benefits universally by citizenship right, in a way that requires high levels of taxation and public expenditure.

This approach demonstrates that social inequalities do not emerge "naturally" from the market, but are instead politically constructed. According to this framework, liberal welfare states such as the United States, the United Kingdom, Canada, Australia, and New Zealand do little to reduce poverty or inequality: wage inequality generated by the labor market is not reduced much, if at all, by fiscal or welfare policy. Conservative welfare states, such as France, Germany, Austria, Italy, and Belgium, provide relatively generous social services and welfare benefits to some statuses of people, but deliver them in ways that reinforce existing patterns of social inequality (e.g., gender roles in the family). Social democratic welfare states, such as Sweden, Denmark, Norway, Finland, and Iceland, reduce poverty and inequality dramatically by providing a wide range of social services. New research has updated and revised Esping-Andersen's regime scheme, contrasting "social market economies" (combining generous social provision with coordinated business interest representation and strong labor unions) with "liberal market economies," with the former outperforming the latter in reducing inequality, without sacrificing economic growth and jobs. For definitions of many of the central terms in the welfare-regimes literature, see Eikemo and Bambra's glossary of welfare-state concepts (Eikemo & Bambra, 2008).

Like the "welfare regimes" approach, the "power constellations" approach theorizes the causes and effects of the welfare state, but here political parties are the central determinant of social welfare policies. Power constellations theory views social democratic parties, Christian Democratic parties, and social movements as engines of distinct welfare-state trajectories, with research demonstrating that party incumbency directly and indirectly affects countries' level and quality of social inequality. While the key causal mechanism in the power constellations approach is the political party, social movements (e.g., labor, feminist, tax-revolt) also play a role in party formation and formal political participation. For instance, power resources theory explains the development of social democratic welfare states as a function of strong labor unions and electorally successful Left parties, both of which served as necessary power resources for the democratic class struggle, in Korpi's famous formulation (Korpi, 1983).

Currently, several European scholars and policymakers advocate a social-investment approach (Esping-Andersen et al., 2002; Midgley, 1999; Morel, Palier, & Palme, 2012). The social-investment approach views the welfare state as investment rather than consumption in macroeconomic terms. Responding to the neoliberal turn in social policymaking in the 1980s and 1990s, advocates for social investment argue for social policy interventions that are most likely to enhance economic productivity, such as early childhood education, pro-family policies such as gender-equitable family leaves, active labor market policies as discussed before, and incentives to include increased participation in the paid labor force. This market-oriented approach to social policy, in contrast to the society-oriented approach of power-resources theory outlined previously, includes new financing channels for social policy expenditure, including social-yield investment bonds.

Beyond typologies, there are two approaches to measuring the welfare state: the institutional approach and the expenditure approach. The institutional approach measures specific citizenship rights as encoded in enacted policies, such as the percentage of one's wages that can be replaced by entitlements such as unemployment insurance, sickness benefits, and public or mandatory private pensions. Such rights are likely to matter for health inequalities because they confer variable control over private goods that give individuals and households power in labor and consumer markets. A common institutional measure of such citizenship rights is the replacement rate, often quantified as the fraction of public benefits to the average per-worker wage. Individual- and household-level replacement rates can be calculated using detailed income surveys, which unfortunately rarely also include measures of health, illness, or mortality. The other major tradition in measuring welfare states is the welfare-effort or expenditure-based approach, which quantifies the extent to which the state makes an effort toward ensuring welfare in different domains by summing the public expenditures in each domain and then dividing that quantity by the size of the eligible population (thus creating an effort-per-capita measure) or by the size of the economy (thus creating a percentage-of-GDP measure). A leading approach to measuring welfare-state characteristics that shape the income distribution is the income-transfers measure (Brady & Bostic, 2015). This measure sums public expenditures across policies that transfer money from the state to individuals and households as income supports, including sickness benefits, pensions, and family supports.

The Comparative Welfare States Dataset (CWS) was one of the earliest contributions to the research infrastructure for comparative political sociology, and was supported by the U.S. National Science Foundation, Northwestern University, and the University of North Carolina–Chapel Hill (Huber et al., 1997). The original scope of this dataset was democratic states in 19 high-income nations, 1960–1998, and it has since been extended to include Greece, Portugal, and Spain, and updated to include later years to 2014 (Brady, Huber, & Stephens, 2016). Variables include wage, salary, and income distribution; public expenditures on many social policies;

policy-based institutional measures of social policy; labor force and labor-market institutions; political coalitions and partisanship of governments; and an array of basic economic and demographic variables.

Inspired by the classic research of Esping-Andersen, the Comparative Welfare Entitlements Dataset (CWED) focuses specifically on social policies that provide rights based on citizenship and thus contribute to the decommodification of labor (Scruggs, 2004). In contrast to the regimes approach, which is helpful for analyzing cross-sectional differences but tends to lump policy domains together, CWED measures include both cross-national and within-nation, over-time variation in welfare states, and program-specific information on the generosity and coverage of unemployment insurance, sickness benefits, and public pension programs. For each program, benefit generosity is measured as a function of (1) the percentage of the average worker wage that is replaced by benefits; (2) the duration of benefits; (3) restrictions on benefit eligibility, such as waiting periods, retirement ages, and work requirements; and (4) the coverage rate or take-up rate. The first three characteristics are each transformed into a z-score, using all available data on each characteristic as the reference distribution. For unemployment insurance and sickness benefits, the relative generosity level of each benefit is then multiplied by the proportion of the labor force that is covered by each benefit. For pensions, the relative generosity is multiplied by the take-up rate. Thus, for each year, and for unemployment, sickness, and pensions, each welfare state receives a generosity score that is based on its benefit generosity relative to the distribution of generosity across all countries and years included in the CWED data, and the extent to which each benefit covers the relevant population. The overall generosity summary score combines this information into one index.

For concreteness, consider the cases of the United States, Germany, and Sweden. In 2010, the United States scored 21.7 on the summary measure of relative generosity, which is mainly a function of low levels of generosity relative to the maximum generosity scores for the countries and years included in the data (maxima on unemployment, sickness, and pensions are observed in Norway 2000–2001, Sweden 1987–1990, and Sweden 1983, respectively). This is toward the low end of summary generosity, which ranged from 20.9 (Australia) to 43.9 (Norway) among the 18 countries in the data in 2010. Germany's summary relative generosity score for 2010 was 32, which is more a function of restricted coverage of non–means-tested public insurance (76% for unemployment insurance, and 83% for sickness insurance) than benefit generosity. In 2010, Sweden's summary relative generosity score was 35.2; its decline from a high of 46.6 in 1989 was a function of declining generosity in all three domains of the welfare state, and declining coverage in the area of unemployment insurance. Crucial for interpretation is the fact that these measures of social policy generosity are inherently relative, although originating in very specific policy indicators. As such, the relative rankings on these measures are reliable, and a one-unit change means the same thing at the bottom of the generosity distribution as it does at the top, but the quantity of each score itself has no direct interpretation (e.g., it is not a percentage). Figures 1.4, 1.5 and 1.6 show how the summary generosity scores have evolved over time for 18 OECD welfare states.

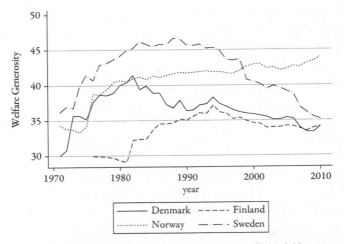

Figure 1.4 *Summary of welfare generosity in Denmark, Finland, Norway, and Sweden, ca. 1970–2010.*

Source: Beckfield, Jason and Clare Bambra. 2016. "Shorter lives in stingier states: Social policy shortcomings help explain the US mortality disadvantage." Social Science & Medicine Volume 171, Pages 30–38.

Note two key characteristics of this summary welfare generosity measure: over-time and cross-national variations, both of which are necessary but not sufficient for identifying institutional effects in quantitative models. Substantively, the retrenchment of the Swedish welfare state is clear in these data, as it reached its maximum in the late 1980s and then began a long, steep decline such that today's Swedish welfare state is no more generous than it was in 1970. This is a striking historical change that has received too little attention in the political-sociology and social epidemiology literatures.

In the conservative welfare states, there is again substantial between-nation and within-nation variation. The average trend

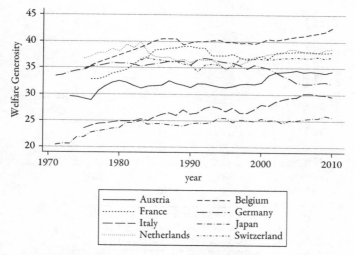

Figure 1.5 *Summary of welfare generosity in Austria, Belgium, France, Germany, Italy, Japan, the Netherlands, and Switzerland, ca. 1970–2010.*

Source: Beckfield, Jason and Clare Bambra. 2016. "Shorter lives in stingier states: Social policy shortcomings help explain the US mortality disadvantage." Social Science & Medicine Volume 171, Pages 30–38.

is moderate growth in generosity over time, with the exceptions of stasis in France and retrenchment in Germany. In Germany, the key welfare-state reforms that yielded this overall retrenchment were reforms to unemployment insurance in the early- to mid-2000s, known as the Hartz reforms after the chair of the commission that designed them. The rising insecurity and stigmatized status of the Hartz benefits have resulted in an unemployment insurance system more similar to that in the United States, with potential consequences for the health of the unemployed in slack labor markets (Noelke & Beckfield, 2014).

In the market-liberal welfare states, the most striking change is the rapid expansion of welfare benefits that followed the "Celtic Tiger"

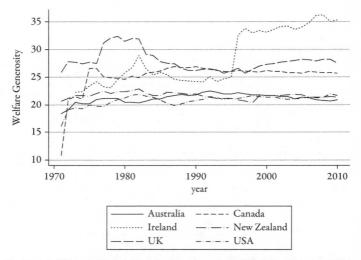

Figure 1.6 *Summary of welfare generosity in Australia, Canada, Ireland, New Zealand, the United Kingdom, and the United States, ca. 1970–2010.*

Source: Beckfield, Jason and Clare Bambra. 2016. "Shorter lives in stingier states: Social policy shortcomings help explain the US mortality disadvantage." *Social Science & Medicine* Volume 171, Pages 30–38.

boom in 1990s Ireland, which demonstrates that economic growth can be broadly distributed depending upon institutional arrangements. Also striking is the long period of retrenchment in the United Kingdom under Thatcher's pro-business and anti-union regime, which further bolsters the historical face-validity of this macroscopic measure. In the United States, overall welfare generosity changed little over the long 1970–2010 period, which matches the historical record of the laggard U.S. welfare state hovering near the bottom rank.

Much of the original source material for these datasets comes from the OECD, which also promotes its preferred social and economic policies, such as the deregulation of labor markets in European welfare states. As ever, politics and science intersect. Through variable lenses, international organizations like the OECD, the International Labor Organization, the United Nations, the World Bank, and the European Union make a wide array of welfare-state measures available. One example is the OECD's *Benefits and Wages* database, which simulates the taxes and benefits owed by or due to people in different family and employment situations, for OECD countries in any given year between 2001 and 2014 (Benefits and Wages: Tax-Benefit Calculator—OECD, n.d.). The National Bureau of Economic Research in the United States offers a taxation simulator, TAXSIM, that calculates the tax burden as well as the value of tax credits under U.S. fiscal policy (Internet TAXSIM Version 9, n.d.). Such information can be combined with the U.S. government's online Social Security benefit calculator, which provides benefit levels back to 1940, when the first pension benefits were paid after the 1935 Social Security Act took effect (Social Security Benefit Calculator Description, n.d.).

The *Luxembourg Income Study* (LIS) and the *Luxembourg Wealth Study* (LWS) are two foundational datasets for the comparative analysis of economic inequality. They are both quite useful for political-sociological analysis, because they allow the analyst to measure redistribution, wage compression, and social welfare receipt directly through comparable, harmonized and (where possible) standardized, individual-level survey data. The LIS project, which started in 1983, established the data infrastructure for a significant turn toward cross-national and over-time comparison in the understanding of what causes income inequality, and now, with the LWS, wealth inequality (Atkinson, Rainwater, & Smeeding, 1995). In the LIS, "harmonization" means organizing data from multiple datasets into a common template, with a common question, and documented response categories. The task at this stage is to document the response categories for all surveys and all years so that they can be evaluated for comparability. "Standardization" in turn refers to ascertaining the extent to which data can be made uniform across surveys for comparative analysis. To accomplish these tasks, the LIS developed novel income concepts that allow for the detailed analysis of the composition of income from various sources, including social programs, across widely varying institutional settings. A key finding of LIS-based research is that welfare states vary greatly in the extent to which they redistribute income, such that the difference between market-income inequality and disposable-income inequality becomes an important axis of institutional variation (Mahler & Jesuit, 2006).

A forefront area of research on the welfare state is the moral configurations that underpin social policy arrangements. The analysis of text data—machine-readable newspaper indices, social media network analysis, and frame analysis—offer researchers opportunities to quantify cultural discourse (Bail, 2014). For instance, Brian Steensland uses discourse analysis of newspaper articles and congressional debates to show how the framing of guaranteed family income plans in the pivotal 1960s and 1970s shifted from a social problems framework to a budgetary framework where fiscal constraints were conceived as exogenous to social policy, and debates over the deserving vs. undeserving poor undermined welfare expansion (Steensland, 2006). A recent double special issue of *Theory and Society* describes several new techniques for measuring culture (Mohr & Ghaziani, 2014), which could be extended to measure the cultural foundations of welfare states. Examples include "productive methods" such as asking Ghanaian respondents to make AIDS posters (T. E. McDonnell, 2014).

Collective Bargaining

Research on economic inequality shows that collective bargaining institutions—corporatist pacts between labor unions, employer organizations, and the state; the occupational structure of wage bargaining; and the organizational strength of labor unions—have some of the strongest effects on changes in inequality over time within countries, and between-country differences at any one point in time. Conceptually, collective bargaining institutions are formal and informal rules that organize power in labor markets. Tripartite corporatist bargaining over employment and wages—classically prominent in many Continental European countries, especially Germany—organizes power in labor markets because it defines whose interests are represented in state-led, sector- or economy-wide negotiations, how those interests are represented, and what settlements over conflicting interests between employees and employers are possible.

Jelle Visser has provided the comparative scholarly community with a powerful data resource for measuring collective bargaining: the Institutional Characteristics of Trade Unions, Wage Setting, State Intervention and Social Pacts (ICTWSS) dataset, which includes annual data on a wide range of measures for 34 countries between the years 1960 and 2007 (Visser, 2011). Union density—the number of union members divided by the number of people in the paid labor force—represents a core, traditional measure of collective bargaining that is often used in comparative research. Contract coverage—the number of workers covered by collective bargaining agreements divided by the number of workers in the paid labor force—represents a complementary measure that allows analysts to account for the fact that in many political-economic contexts, such as France, workers are covered by collective bargaining agreements even when they are not members of any union.

Figure 1.7 depicts changing collective bargaining institutions, as measured by union density, for several high-income countries of the OECD (Pinto & Beckfield, 2011).

What stands out from the figure is a decline in unionization in several national political economies, especially after the 1980s.

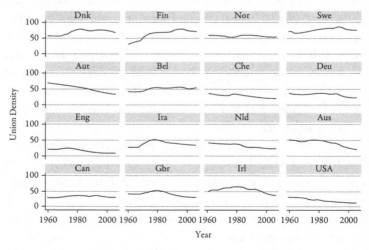

Figure 1.7 *Union density in 16 rich democracies, 1960–2007.*

Source: Pinto, Sanjay and Jason Beckfield. 2011. "Organized Labor in an Evolving Europe." Research in the Sociology of Work 22:153–179.

Given the importance of collective bargaining institutions for the power that workers possess in labor markets, it seems possible that this changing institutional context might shape the changing distribution of population health. For instance, as union membership grows rarer, it might become a more important social determinant of health. It could also be the case that union decline contributes to the U.S. mortality disadvantage relative to rich democracies with stronger collective bargaining institutions.

Policy Domains

A policy domain, or field, is a substantive collection of people and organizations with common interests in a given area of policymaking. The substance that defines the field and sets its boundaries is the object of policy: for instance, health care is a large policy domain in many rich democracies that includes interested policymakers, public healthcare employees, medical organizations, hospital organizations, public health scholars and activists, and other constituencies with a stake in healthcare. Other policy domains include environmental regulation, energy, immigration, pensions, agriculture, education, and labor; each has its distinctive organizational structure and substantive conflicts.

Of course, the boundaries of a policy domain are contested, as incumbents and challengers seek to gain advantage through rewriting the rules of the game. Such dynamics are well conceptualized by field analysis, an area of scholarship that includes cultural sociology, economic sociology, political sociology, and the sociology of organizations (Fligstein, 2001; Fligstein & McAdam, 2012). The health policy domain is easily the most investigated by social epidemiologists, so it warrants a detailed discussion here.

Indeed, healthcare policy is the substantive area of greatest overlap between social epidemiology, medical sociology, and political sociology (D. Cutler, 2004; McKeown, 2014 [1979]; McKinlay & McKinlay, 1977).

Research on comparative healthcare systems connects the interests of social epidemiologists, who might investigate healthcare utilization, and political sociologists, who might investigate cross-national or sub-national regional differences in health policy and healthcare systems (Beckfield, Olafsdottir, & Sosnaud, 2013; Lynch, 2008). In one of the first attempts to test empirically how healthcare systems cluster, Wendt (2009) analyzed 15 European healthcare systems to construct groups of healthcare systems. The cluster analysis identified unique combinations of expenditure, financing, service provision, and access regulation. Using the broad categories of health expenditure and private payment, healthcare provider indices, and institutional indicators, he identified three distinctive healthcare types: the health service provision–oriented type, the universal coverage–controlled access type, and the low budget–restricted access type.

Austria, Belgium, France, Germany, and Luxembourg exemplify the health service provision–oriented type. These systems prioritize service provision, especially in the outpatient sector. There are many providers, and patients have relatively free choice among medical doctors. Patients are expected to pay only a modest out-of-pocket copayment. Importantly, and in contrast to the United States, autonomy of patients and equal access are greatly valued and weigh more heavily than the autonomy of the medical profession. Denmark, Great Britain, Sweden, Italy, and Ireland represent the universal coverage–controlled access type. Here, all citizens are covered through universal plans, but access to care is more strictly regulated by the state. Finally, Portugal, Spain, and Finland comprise the low budget–restricted access type. Healthcare spending in these systems is comparatively low, and system usage is restricted through high copayments and requirements that patients use the same doctor over time. Key sources of data on health policy domains, of which healthcare systems form a crucial component, are available from NGOs such as the Commonwealth Fund, which collects rich comparative cross-national data. Intergovernmental Organizations (IGOs) such as the World Health Organization also provide system-level data, including financing and expenditure data from the System of Health Accounts. Electronic health records, such as those available from public clinics in China, and Medicaid and Medicare data in the United States, are emerging sources of information on healthcare systems.

Mobilization

Political participation, or the direct engagement in political processes by members of a polity, is often separated into formal and informal participation. "Formal political participation" means membership in political organizations or parties, lobbying powerful actors through channels of interest representation, voting for candidates in elections, and standing for election. "Informal political participation" is often conceptualized as various forms, variably organized, of "street politics" outside the formal organization of the state.

In the discipline of sociology, research on collective behavior and social movements is one of the largest subfields, and overlaps with political sociology in its investigation of the organization and reorganization of power through engagement with the state from within and without. "Contestation" refers to organized conflict over a given issue, from free trade agreements as in the anti-WTO Seattle protests, to financial power in the Occupy Wall Street protests, to labor relations in the French protests over a neoliberal labor law in the summer of 2016, to ongoing protests over migrants in Europe, to protests against the Trump administration in the United States. "Mobilization" refers to the social processes whereby people constitute a social movement, often through social movement organizations or social media (Davis, McAdam, Scott, & Zald, 2005).

A theoretically plausible, direct link from mobilization to population health is the social interaction and social support that mobilization can generate; another is feedback effects from population health problems to the political system. There are several empirical approaches toward studying social movements. A classic is the survey, as used for McAdam's *Freedom Summer* study of the US Civil Rights Movement (McAdam, 1990). Other scholars conduct ethnographic and interview-based research in revolutionary-war contexts (Viterna, 2013). Still others conduct historical-sociological analysis based on archival data, e.g. of the organizational roles of Black churches in the US Civil Rights Movement (Morris, 1981). Social-media data are also used to analyze social movements in rich democracies, including the Black Lives Matter movement in the US, which responds to racialized police violence (Earl & Kimport, 2011; Ray et al., 2017). In drawing out the connections between social mobilization and population health, it may be useful to distinguish between (1) mobilization around a health issue and its potential effects on that issue, (2) general mobilization which may have general health effects through framing historical trauma as a public problem rather than an individual failing, and (3) mobilization that begins with a health issue (e.g. HIV and AIDS in the US in the 1980s) and may then contribute to wider societal effects (e.g. liberalization of state regulations of same-sex sexual relations in the US and elsewhere).

Public Opinion

The role of public opinion in democratic politics is contested, with debate over whether public opinion is better conceptualized as a cause or an effect of policymaking. One argument for public opinion as a cause of policy comes from dynamic representation theory, which holds that policymakers are disciplined by the electoral system: public preferences shape policy through changing partisan composition of government, and elected policymakers anticipate electoral gains and losses from policy choices. In both cases, changes in aggregate preferences of the public toward policy choices are associated with changes in enacted policies (Stimson, Mackuen, & Erikson, 1995). On the other hand, public opinion often follows policy changes, as policies create their own constituencies (Brooks & Manza, 2008). A key insight from historical institutionalists is that the processes producing feedback between public opinion and public policy are historically contingent and themselves vary according to institutional arrangements such as electoral systems and the organization of democratic representation (Pierson, 1993, 2004).

Whether public opinion is cause, effect, or both, the partisan composition of a government is a key political-sociological mechanism. In democratic polities where interests are represented for the purposes of elections through organizations we call political parties, the partisanship of a government denotes the location of the party or parties (in the case of coalitions in proportional representation systems) in power. Often, for the purpose of measurement, parties are arrayed on a left-center-right ideological spectrum, on the basis of expert surveys or party manifestos, although there is debate about the utility of the left–right continuum for capturing symbolic politics in domains defined by identity, recognition, and the environment (Häusermann, 2006; Häusermann & Kriesi, 2011). Focusing more on politics than on policies are the Comparative Political Data Set (CPDS) I, II, and III. For the set of rich democracies, plus the new member states of the European Union and select other polities, the CPDSs include a rich array of partisanship measures for executive cabinets and parliaments, along with coalition data. Few studies to date link partisanship to population health (Rodriguez, Bound, & Geronimus, 2014). The computational analysis of textual data also enables quantitative analysis of political discourse, offering opportunities to measure public opinion in a more dynamic and disaggregated way (Bail, 2014).

2 | NEW QUESTIONS AND ANSWERS ABOUT EMBODIED SOCIAL INEQUALITIES

How might the political-sociological concepts reviewed in the last chapter contribute to the distribution of population health? To connect the dots, I begin this chapter with a reconsideration of several established facts about social inequalities in health. Next, I discuss new evidence that establishes relationships between political-sociological structures and processes described in the last chapter, and social inequalities in health. Table 2.1 summarizes the evidence. Because research on the political-sociological foundations of health distribution is a relatively new area, not every political "exposure" listed in Table 1.1 appears in Table 2.1.

Disease is distributed unequally within populations according to socioeconomic position (SEP), even after controlling for the many behavioral and other factors that affect health and are also—variably across institutional contexts—correlated with SEP, like diet, exercise, smoking, excessive drinking, and healthcare access. One of the strongest demonstrations of this gradient appeared in the work of Michael Marmot and collaborators, who discovered a very steep health gradient even among male public employees working in

Table 2.1 **Key Studies Relevant to the Political Sociology of Health Inequalities**

Evidence	Study Population	Potential Exposure
1. Employment grade is associated with death from CVD	U.K. male civil servants	Institutions of Employment
2. Deaths from CVD cluster in the states of the American South	U.S. adults aged 35+	Polity; Federalism
3. Infant mortality rates are distributed unequally across sub-national areas across the world	Recorded live births	World Polity; Nation-State; Political Economy
4. The prevalence of and inequality in poor self-rated health are unrelated	U.S. adults	State-Level Social Policy
5. Public health expenditure reduces the effect of household wealth on under-five mortality	34 low-income nations	Welfare State; Public Health Policy
6. Educational expansion reduces the effect of maternal education on under-five mortality	34 low-income nations	Welfare State; Education Policy
7. Dismantlement of racial subordination policies reduces infant mortality rates	U.S. live births	Political Incorporation

Table 2.1 Continued

Evidence	Study Population	Potential Exposure
8. Skin color relates to self-perceived discrimination and self-rated health in the United States	Native-born U.S. black adults	Racial Formation
9. Social policies of the welfare state reduce health penalties of lone-parenthood and poverty	High-income countries	Welfare State; Gendered State
10. Social protection (unemployment benefits and labor regulations) reduce mortality among women	High-income countries	Welfare State; Gendered State
11. Income inequality strengthens the effect of income on health, raising health inequality	World Values Survey samples	Political Economy
12. Neoliberal economic reforms increase health inequalities	U.K., Australia, New Zealand	Political Economy
13. The transition to capitalism increased inequalities in mortality	Central and Eastern Europe	Political Economy
14. Union membership enhances self-rated health	U.S. 1973–2006	Collective Bargaining

Whitehall (the British civil service) in London. As the now-famous evidence from their Whitehall Study shows, men embodied their stratified positions within the organizational hierarchy in multiple ways, including coronary heart disease, as shown in Figure 2.1.

Again, for U.S.-based readers, it is important to underscore the fact that all these civil servants had access to healthcare through the National Health Service (NHS), which was founded in 1948. The gradient in these data also appeared even after controlling

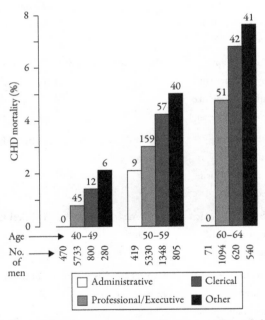

Figure 2.1 *The gradient in coronary heart disease mortality risk by occupational rank in the British civil service, as reported by the Whitehall Study.*

Source: Marmot MG, Rose G, Shipley M, et al. Employment grade and coronary heart disease in British civil servants. Journal of Epidemiology & Community Health 1978; 32:244–249.

for the usual behavioral suspects or their rough proxies (cholesterol, smoking, exercise, and other factors), as Figure 2.2 shows. Strikingly, civil servants working in the lower employment grades were 2.1, 3.2, and 4.0 times as likely as civil servants working in the top employment grade to die by heart attack. Most of these inequities were unexplained by the many biomedical and behavioral factors Marmot's group measured and included in the

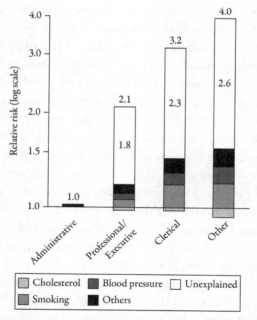

Figure 2.2 *Explained and unexplained components of the gradient in coronary heart disease mortality risk by occupational rank in the British civil service, as reported by the Whitehall Study.*

Source: Marmot MG, Rose G, Shipley M, et al. Employment grade and coronary heart disease in British civil servants. Journal of Epidemiology & Community Health 1978; 32:244–249.

models; later work also investigated early-life exposures (Smith, Shipley, & Rose, 1990).

How does a consideration of political sociology help us to explain these facts? First, politics and policies affect the selection of people into the organization. Employment laws and regulations at the macro level shape the kinds of qualifications available to people, and in what quality and quantity. Such institutional arrangements also shape the quantity and quality of organizational discretion in hiring, compensation, work autonomy, and termination practices. These institutionalized processes play out over the lifecourse, from one's birth into a household with social and economic resources, to one's neighborhood and schooling opportunities, to one's own family formation. And so, in considering the people who populate this figure and the Whitehall data, we must think about the institutional contexts they embody as they are selected by powerful others for varying levels of educational certification, occupational licensure, organizational power, and unequal remuneration. That is, macroscopic political-sociological factors have selected some people over others for stratified and organized positions, and in that sense the health gradient can be over-determined by the dual influence of institutional selection and institutionalized hierarchy. For instance, the Whitehall Study in fact massively under-estimated the magnitude of health inequities in the U.K. population, given the selectivity of civil servants, the inclusion of only males, and the single-variable measurement of SEP (Smith et al., 1990). Moreover, the political-sociological context also shapes the distribution of resources that matter for health (in this case, the size and number of occupational grades that take on social significance and are embodied in the form of differential cardiovascular disease [CVD] mortality), the processes whereby the social determinants of health generate health and disease, and the other resources that stratified organizational positions bring (cf. Kelly, 1980).

Of course, while political sociology embeds and helps to interpret in new ways the classic Whitehall results, this example limits the political sociological perspective because the range of institutional variation is necessarily and intentionally truncated in the study of British civil servants. That is, Marmot and collaborators observed within one nation-state (indeed, one city) over a relatively limited time span (later extended, by Whitehall II). What this means is that several institutional factors—potential causes of health inequities—are held constant in the Whitehall Study, and so cannot emerge from the analysis as causes. But if we broaden our political-geographic scope, we can explore the role of other political-sociological factors, including variable political incorporation, social policy, gendered state, health care, and labor market arrangements. Consider the 50 United States. Often in comparative research, the United States is treated as one case, but this elides substantial within-U.S. variation that is itself politically rooted—in federalism. Figure 2.3 below from the U.S. Centers for Disease Control and Prevention (CDC) shows that state-level factors probably contribute to the large variation among U.S. counties in cardiovascular mortality. The sickest counties, which cluster in Oklahoma, Missouri, Arkansas, Louisiana, Kentucky, Tennessee, Alabama, Mississippi, and Georgia, have CVD mortality rates from 4 to 10 times higher than the healthiest counties'.

In Figure 2.3, adults aged 35 and over living in U.S. counties at the time of data collection have widely varying rates of death

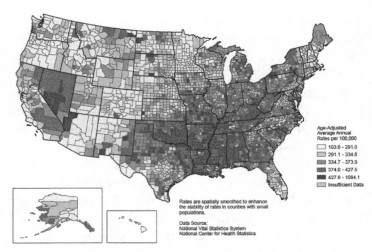

Figure 2.3 *Heart disease death rates in the United States, adults ages 35+, by county, 2011–2013.*

Source: https://www.cdc.gov/dhdsp/maps/national_maps/hd_all.htm

due to CVD, and these rates imperfectly correspond to political lines drawn by the federal structure of the United States. For instance, states with relatively homogeneous rates of CVD mortality are apparent in the figure—e.g. Nevada, Alabama, and Mississippi with homogeneously high rates, and Oregon, Colorado, and Massachusetts with homogeneously low rates. But the predominant pattern in the map of CVD mortality in U.S. counties is that clusters of high and low CVD mortality are not contained by the political boundaries of states. Some of these spillovers probably result from ecological conditions that may be politically driven, but nevertheless cross state boundaries, such as the legacy of Jim Crow in the southern Black Belt, the mining industry in Appalachia, the petroleum industry in Texas and Oklahoma, and deindustrialization in the Rust Belt. Some spillovers probably also result from interstate migration, as mobile people carry political contexts with them throughout the lifecourse. Nevertheless, in thinking about the pattern of CVD mortality distribution across the United States, with a concentration of high levels in the American South, it seems reasonable that the troubled history of racial politics in the United States probably plays an important role, as the Jim Crow system of racial exclusion and oppression did follow state lines (Krieger et al., 2013). Such political-sociological arrangements can be systematically conceptualized and measured, as the last chapter detailed.

Because economic segregation is high and growing in the United States, it is possible to use information on the socioeconomic attributes of small geographic aggregates such as census blocks, tracts, and counties to gain leverage on the economic distribution of mortality within each of the 50 states (Reardon & Bischoff, 2011). One would prefer to have household- and individual-level data on income and mortality for a sufficiently large sample of individuals in the United States to allow for within-state analyses across all 50 states, but at present such data simply do not exist (Krieger, 2011). Using county income quintile as a proxy for the economic position of people living in counties, previous work shows that economic inequality in mortality within states varies greatly between states: in some states, it matters a lot whether one lives in a rich or poor county, while in others it matters much less. Moreover, aggregate U.S.-level health inequality between rich and poor counties trends nonlinearly since 1960, declining until the 1980s, then increasing in the 1990s and through the 2000s. This raises the crucial conceptual point that, in analyzing population health, it is essential to differentiate the distribution from the central tendency. That is, even as aggregate-average population health is improving, inequalities can rise or decline (Krieger et al., 2008).

Figure 2.4 makes this point in a striking way, using U.S. data. This figure shows clearly the non-relationship between aggregate-average population health on the one hand, and inequality in the distribution of population health on the other. For this analysis of the average health of the 50 U.S. states, and health inequality within each of the 50 states, it was necessary to use survey data on self-rated health instead of CVD mortality data, since the necessary data are simply unavailable for CVD mortality, or even

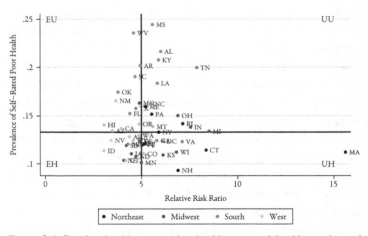

Figure 2.4 *Equal unhealthy, unequal unhealthy, unequal healthy, and equal healthy States of the Union, ca. 2008–2010.*

Source: Beckfield, Jason and Katherine Morris. 2016. "Health (a report on health inequalities in the US for the annual 'State of the Union' issue)." Pathways. Stanford Center on Poverty and Inequality.

all-cause mortality. Self-rated health is surprisingly strongly correlated with mortality risk, physician-diagnosed conditions, and
other objective measures of health, but it has limitations just like
any other single measure (Idler & Benyamini, 1997; Quesnel–
Vallée, 2007). The figure shows that the prevalence of poor self-
rated health in a state (a measure of aggregate-average state health)
is not associated with the degree of dispersion in the distribution
of poor self-rated health across the people living in a state. This
supports the conceptual point that, in understanding population
health, we must separate its average level in the population (however defined) from its distribution within that population.

This conceptual point only gains in significance as we zoom
farther out in the analysis of global health inequality. Certainly
one can treat the global human population as the relevant unit of
analysis and measure change over time in average health or health
inequality (Goesling & Firebaugh, 2004). Such an approach could
be called a "global ecology of population health." This would raise
difficulties for a political-sociological analysis, though, given the
severe measurement and inferential challenges to the identification of global institutional causes. Arguably more promising for
the political sociology of population health, we can define the unit
of analysis according to the unit of political exposure. That is, in
developing and testing hypotheses about the political-sociological
distributors of population health, the political geography of the
relevant exposure can define the unit of analysis, locate causation,
and identify remedies (Krieger et al., 2013; Lynch, 2008).

The global distribution of population health supports a de-
nationalized approach in many regions of the world (Sassen, 2006).
Consider, for example, the distribution of infant mortality. Figures 2.5
and 2.6 show the distribution of infant mortality across nation-states,

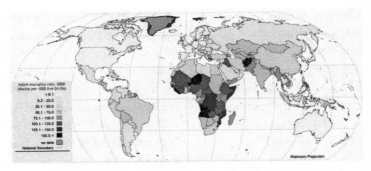

Figure 2.5 *Infant mortality rates within national boundaries, ca. 2000.*

Source: Storeygard, A., Balk, D., Levy, M. and Deane, G. (2008), The global distribution of infant mortality: a subnational spatial view. Popul. Space Place, 14: 209–229. doi:10.1002/psp.484

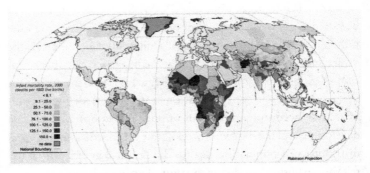

Figure 2.6 *Infant mortality rates in small geographic areas (roughly counties), ca. 2000.*

Source: Storeygard, A., Balk, D., Levy, M. and Deane, G. (2008), The global distribution of infant mortality: a subnational spatial view. Popul. Space Place, 14: 209–229. doi:10.1002/psp.484

followed by the distribution of infant mortality across county-sized or smaller areas (Storeygard, Balk, Levy, & Deane, 2008).

In these figures, the internal heterogeneity of the larger countries stands out. For instance, higher infant mortality rates in the American South appear, as do higher infant mortality rates in rural China, northern and eastern Brazil, northern India, South Africa away from Cape Town, and poorer parts of India. Likewise, areas of striking homogeneity appear, including the low-mortality regime encompassing many Western European nations (though there are still deep social inequalities in health in European populations; for a compelling analysis, see Mackenbach, 2013). From a global perspective, then, the striking thing about the distribution of health is the large amount of inequality we observe, with the lowest rates of infant mortality below 9 deaths per 1,000 live births, and the highest rates of infant mortality close to 150 deaths per live births. Also striking is the geographical concentration of global infant mortality in just a few parts of Africa and South Asia.

Since the higher-mortality places shown in the world maps just mentioned are some of the poorest places in the world, and since poverty and inequality are strongly associated, readers might be tempted to infer that health inequality and average health go together. New comparative cross-national and longitudinal research on the distribution of population health in high-mortality countries suggests that this inference would be as incorrect in the Global South as it is in the United States (Sosnaud & Beckfield, 2017). Instead, there is emerging evidence that institutions—of political incorporation, welfare states, and collective bargaining—contribute to the distribution of population health in ways that decouple health inequality from average population health. For instance, public health investment can weaken the link between household wealth and under-five mortality (Sosnaud & Beckfield, 2017).

Political Incorporation and Racial Formation

In the United States, a major axis of political exclusion is race, which itself can be understood as a system of categorization that rests on politics, policy, and law, given that there is no genotypical or phenotypical basis for stable racial classification. Instead, racial classification follows racial formation projects, and the "color line" varies by place and time rather than by people (Omi & Winant, 2014). Indeed, even the classification of the same individuals by observers varies according to changes in employment, social status, and incarceration, which are racialized in the United States (Saperstein & Penner, 2012). While a large literature in social epidemiology establishes that racism and discrimination hurt health, the potential roles of political incorporation in reducing racial inequities in health are less understood.

The timing of dismantling Jim Crow—the system of racial oppression that supported *de jure* segregation in healthcare facilities and other nominally public facilities and maintained a *de facto* system of exclusion from voting through poll tests and taxes in many states of the United States before the Civil Rights Acts of 1964 and 1965—offers analysts opportunities to test hypotheses about political incorporation effects on health. Figure 2.7 shows results from one such study, which examined infant mortality—a health outcome with a relatively short etiologic period responsive to changing social conditions—as a function of race–polity combinations, in an attempt to measure the political-institutional

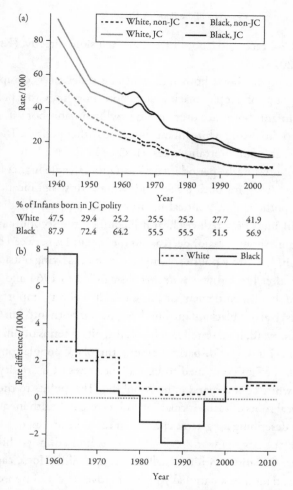

Figure 2.7 *The dismantlement of Jim Crow is associated with declining racial health inequities in the United States, 1940–2010.*

Source: Krieger, Nancy, Jarvis T Chen, Brent Coull, Pamela D Waterman and Jason Beckfield. 2013. "The Unique Impact of Abolition of Jim Crow Laws on Reducing Inequities in Infant Death Rates and Implications for Choice of Comparison Groups in Analyzing Social Determinants of Health." *American Journal of Public Health* 103:2234–2244.

reality of race and roots of racial exclusion directly (Krieger et al., 2013).

The figure shows both rates and rate differences, comparing four groups of people: black infants born into Jim Crow polities, black infants born into other polities, white infants born into Jim Crow polities, and white infants born into other polities. The data show that infant mortality rates fell since 1940 for all groups, and that for most of the period infant mortality rates are higher in Jim Crow polities, for both blacks and whites. Most significantly for the hypothesis that political incorporation through the dismantling of Jim Crow reduces health inequities, the second panel in the figure shows a major decrease in the inequities between blacks living in Jim Crow polities, compared to blacks living outside Jim Crow, after Jim Crow was *de jure* dismantled in 1964 and 1965. Before the dismantlement of Jim Crow, it was very important to the survival of a black infant whether s/he was born into Jim Crow, but afterward, it mattered much less, if at all, in terms of Jim Crow vs. non–Jim Crow disparities among the black population, even as both groups continued to have higher rates of mortality than their white counterparts in both polities. This points to the clear political roots of racial formation and its role in health inequities.

In describing long-term changes in racial health inequities, research such as the work reviewed here is limited in its ability to capture variation within racialized groups. Ellis Monk captures such variation in a nationally representative survey of households with at least one African American over the age of 18; this survey includes interviewer and respondent ratings of skin color, allowing Monk to investigate the health impact of colorism and embodied racialized status. He finds that darker skin color is positively associated with discrimination reported by African Americans, in everyday interactions with both blacks and whites. This discrimination, in turn, is negatively associated with self-rated physical and mental health. This evidence supports the inference that processes of racial formation—strongly linked to skin color in the U.S. system of racial differentiation—contribute to the stratification of health outcomes. It remains an open question whether other axes of racial categorization in other parts of the world are similarly associated with everyday discrimination and its health consequences, though this is an active area of research, especially on colorism in Brazil (Monk, 2016). Such comparative institutional research can help to reveal how race is constituted by variable and thus modifiable institutional arrangements.

For example, Dong Han argues that rural migrant status is racialized in China through policing practices of the Chinese state (D. Han, 2010). The institution of *hukou*—rural to urban migrant—status in China plays a role in distributing health. Indeed, there is a debate over whether and how rural/urban sociopolitical status may be changing as a social determinant of health in China, as China undergoes a period of rapid economic change. For instance, Song and Burgard find that rural/urban status is a durable determinant of infant mortality in China, with the effect of this status largely undisturbed in China over the long and dynamic 1970–2001 period (Song & Burgard, 2008). For self-rated health, Chen, Yang, and Liu find stark inter-cohort differences within urban and rural populations, with growing gradients by income and education for rural Chinese, net of cohort differences (Chen, Yang, & Liu, 2010). Using data on both self-rated physical and mental health, Whyte and Tsang (forthcoming) find that rural Chinese actually reported their own health as better in 2004, but worse in 2014 after significant health-insurance reforms.

Of the studies reviewed by myself and Krieger (Beckfield & Krieger, 2009), two reported that the dismantling of apartheid in post-1990 South Africa was not associated with reductions in racial/ethnic inequities in physical growth in infancy or infant mortality, although a third found that extending the comparative timeframe back to 1970 showed that racial/ethnic disparities in South African infant and child mortality had in fact declined. In the case of indigenous populations, research in New Zealand found that Maori–European relative and absolute health inequities widened following neoliberal reforms, and also that Aboriginal health disparities in Australia grew during a period of policy inattention. Detailed cross-national case comparison of HIV/AIDS policy in Brazil vs. South Africa shows that "boundary institutions" that cement group differences in law, policy, and organizations of the state hindered the development of collective efforts to address the population health crisis in South Africa, but not in Brazil, where group boundaries are colorized but not racialized, and "whitening" is institutionalized (Gauri & Lieberman, 2006). Such institutionalization could be conceptualized as one form of civic stratification (Torres & Waldinger, 2015), where the common thread is political incorporation and exclusion.

Welfare States in the Global South

As under-five mortality rates decline in the Global South, inequality according to household wealth and maternal education tend to decline. These declines in inequity cut against the grain of research suggesting that health inequalities should grow or at least remain stable as population health improves (D. M. Cutler, Deaton, & Lleras-Muney, 2006; Link & Phelan, 1995). Instead, declines in health inequalities by education and wealth are systematically steeper in nations where national policies are more inclusive of women in formal schooling, and distribute more resources for public health (Sosnaud & Beckfield, 2017). Later in this chapter, I summarize the arguments and evidence for health-inequality-reducing effects of two significant welfare-state institutions in low- and middle-income countries: public health infrastructure and educational expansion. The political sociology here is in the identification and testing of hypotheses about public health investment and educational expansion as political choices that stratify the population, as well as affect the effects of stratification. Political sociology thus identifies the welfare state as a double cause of embodied social inequality.

The argument for the role of the public health infrastructure—an institutional variable and part of the welfare state—in reducing inequality in under-five mortality in low-income countries begins with the strong association between household economic resources and child health outcomes (Sosnaud & Beckfield, 2017). The association between family SEP and child health outcomes in developing nations has been shown to reflect a multitude of pathways and mechanisms. One key pathway involves the role of economic resources in structuring a child's exposure to more proximate health determinants like proper nutrition, medical treatment, and safe housing. Due to the lack of reliable and comparable data on household income, studies of health inequalities in developing countries rely on wealth as the primary measure of material resources. Wealth indices based on asset ownership capture a family's ability to obtain health-promoting goods and services, and account for resources obtained from informal employment relationships. Research demonstrates a significant and positive association between household wealth and child health in developing nations, though the strength of this association varies across national contexts, raising questions about what institutional variables increase and decrease inequality.

Public health expenditure represents an institutional variable that can reduce social inequality in health by weakening the link between private material resources and health outcomes. For example, the construction of new hospitals and health clinics represents a key source of government health spending in developing countries. If this expenditure promotes more universal usage of quality medical care, immunizations, and other treatments, then household economic resources may become less important in determining which children receive these services.

Sosnaud and I (Sosnaud & Beckfield, 2017) investigated this question of how public health expenditure, a welfare-state measure appropriate to low- and middle-income countries with high under-five mortality rates caused by diseases readily amenable to treatment, contributes to inequities in under-five mortality by household wealth and maternal education. Figures 2.8–2.11 show evidence from this study: the first two figures show that as overall under-five mortality rates decline, wealth- and education-based inequalities in the chance that a child dies before the age of five decline, rather than rise (as calculated from data across the 1990–2011 period, from demographic surveys conducted between 1995 and 2016, as well as national vital statistics). The third figure shows that public health expenditure—publicly guided expenditures of resources from domestic and international sources on, for instance, vaccination programs, community health workers, free or low-cost medications, and transportation to medical facilities—does moderate the relationship between household wealth and the chance that a child dies before the age of five. The fourth figure shows that educational expansion—an institutional cause of the decline in educational stratification—reduces inequities in under-five mortality by maternal education.

Specifically, Figure 2.8 shows that instead of increasing inequality with declining under-five mortality, inequality in the

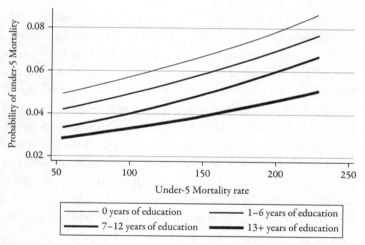

Figure 2.8 *Inequity in under-five mortality by maternal education declines as overall under-five mortality rate declines.*

Source: Sosnaud and Beckfield (2017), Journal of Health and Social Behavior. Original data are from various sources, including the Demographic & Health Surveys.

chance of death before the age of five based on the mother's educational attainment decreased in these countries. Importantly, these estimates are based on fixed-effects estimation that removes the effects of durable between-country differences that can undermine cross-national comparability. So, we can infer from the figure that within-country improvements over time in prevailing mortality conditions are associated with within-country reductions in the extent to which maternal education matters for child survival. Specifically, the gap between babies born to the highest-educated mothers and less-educated mothers is what drives the decrease in inequality. It is the advantage of the highest level of schooling that decreases in these low-income countries.

Figure 2.9 shows that the decrease in mortality inequality while mortality declines is not limited to the axis of maternal education. Rather, it generalizes to household wealth: in these low-income countries, as mortality declines it becomes less important whether a baby is born into a wealthy or a poor household. The big advantage of wealth, observed at under-five mortality rates of over 200 per 1,000 live births, decreases as the under-five mortality rate drops below 100 per 1,000 live births. These declines apply to the differences between wealthier households in the top quintile, as compared to the second quintile, third quintile, fourth quintile, and fifth quintile. Interestingly, the distinctive disadvantage of being born into a household in the bottom of the national wealth distribution seems to grow as the national rate of under-five mortality declines.

There is evidence that public-health expenditures in the low-income nations examined here moderate the relationship between wealth and under-five mortality, such that mortality inequality is reduced by public-health expenditure, which might substitute for private wealth through the provision of public goods.

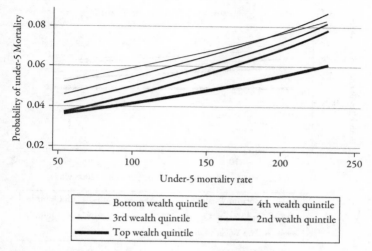

Figure 2.9 *Inequity in under-five mortality by household wealth declines as overall under-five mortality rate declines.*

Source: Sosnaud and Beckfield (2017), Journal of Health and Social Behavior. Original data are from various sources, including the Demographic & Health Surveys.

Figure 2.10 shows evidence from the same study of social inequalities in under-five mortality.

While it is always better for an infant in these low-income countries, regardless of the level of public health spending, to be born into a wealthier household, public health expenditures influence how much better it is. The gap between the top wealth quintile and all the lower quintiles, in terms of the chance of under-five mortality, is smallest where public health expenditure per capita is greatest. While we currently lack the sort of data that would be needed to evaluate the interactions involved between people in these low-income countries and their public health systems, the

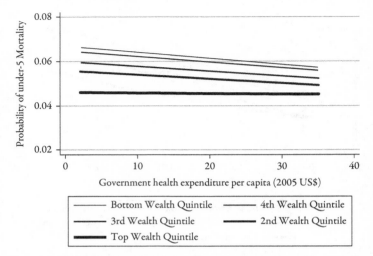

Figure 2.10 *Public (government) health expenditure per capita reduces inequities in under-five mortality by household wealth.*

Source: Sosnaud and Beckfield (2017), Journal of Health and Social Behavior. Original data are from various sources, including the Demographic & Health Surveys.

evidence supports a scenario wherein public health can substitute for private wealth.

Sosnaud and I (Sosnaud & Beckfield, 2017) also investigated the spread of education as a macroscopic institutional variable that moderates the advantage to children of being born to a mother with a higher level of educational attainment. Numerous studies highlight a relationship between maternal education and child health, and evidence suggests that education provides both health knowledge and high-order cognitive skills that increase the use of health services and promote practices that benefit child well-being. Although maternal education is also a proxy for household

economic standing, studies that account for both maternal education and household wealth suggest that these factors are independently associated with child health and mortality.

Educational expansion can shape inequalities in under-five mortality by changing the distribution of socioeconomic resources in developing nations. Systems of formal schooling have been expanding
since the "third wave" of democratization in the 1970s, and the
incorporation of women into these systems has increased dramatically in many developing nations. For example, in Ethiopia, the
percentage of women obtaining at least some primary or secondary
education by age 18 increased from 35% to 83% between 1990 and
2006. If this growth primarily benefits those who had previously
faced barriers to formal schooling, then educational expansion can
be expected to produce a more equal distribution of socioeconomic
resources. As more women gain access to the social and economic
benefits of educational attainment, this is likely to reduce disparities
in the assets, skills, and information that matter for child health. If
so, then differences in under-five mortality by maternal education
can be expected to decline as access to education expands.

Figure 2.11 shows data that support the educational equal-
ization hypothesis: as educational systems expand in the same
low-income countries examined in the section on public health
expenditure, the effect of maternal education shrinks.

Specifically, as the percentage of women in a given national
population who have attained a primary or secondary level of
formal schooling grows, in part as a result of political decisions
to expand access to formal schooling, mortality inequality by maternal education shrinks. In other words, educational expansion
makes it less important whether a baby's mother is more or less formally schooled. The reduction in inequality appears to be driven

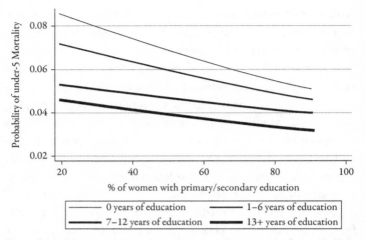

Figure 2.11 *Educational expansion reduces inequities in under-five mortality by maternal educational attainment.*

Source: Sosnaud and Beckfield (2017), Journal of Health and Social Behavior. Original data are from various sources, including the Demographic & Health Surveys.

by stronger decreases in the disadvantages of the lowest levels of formal educational attainment. Theoretically, what this suggests is that institutional arrangements, which shape the structure of social stratification itself, matter for the distribution of health across stratified societies.

Welfare States in the Global North

In one of the first review essays on the relationship between political institutions and health inequities, Krieger and I (Beckfield

& Krieger, 2009) identified 23 studies of the implications of the welfare state for health inequity. They offered deeply divergent findings. Underscoring the possibility of different welfare-state effects on health inequities, these 23 studies produce three themes: (1) the effect of the health system itself on health inequities; (2) the effect of welfare state policy domains that lie outside health insurance, the medical system, and public health; and (3) the effect of welfare regime type on health inequities.

Among the nine studies of the effect of the health-policy domain within the welfare state, five provided evidence that enhancement of welfare state provisions reduced relative health inequities. Two used Canadian data linking the establishment of national health insurance to decreased income-based relative inequities in mortality due to conditions amenable to medical treatment. However, one study of the establishment of the Australian national health care system found that it was simultaneously associated with increased relative—but decreased absolute—socioeconomic inequalities in avoidable mortality. A study of the introduction of freely available, highly active antiretroviral therapy in Barcelona, Spain, observed that education-based inequality in AIDS mortality remained stable. Additionally, two studies focused on Western Europe, where the welfare state has seen its most advanced expression, reported that enhancement of welfare state health systems did not translate to reduced health inequities: one in Norway, on post-neonatal mortality, and one comparing class inequality in infant mortality in the United Kingdom and Sweden.

Conversely, among the 11 European and U.S. studies concerned with whether welfare-state policies outside the health domain counteract the effects of the market and other social forces in producing health inequality, five found evidence that strong welfare states and generous social policies can dampen social inequities in health. For instance, a study using U.S. data found that relative and absolute socioeconomic inequities in premature mortality and infant mortality, especially among populations of color, were at their lowest following the 1960s "War on Poverty," the enactment of civil rights legislation, and the growth of the U.S. welfare state, with these gains reversed in subsequent neoliberal reforms (Krieger et al., 2008). Likewise, Olafsdottir (2007) found that current relative socioeconomic inequalities in self-rated health are lower in social democratic Iceland compared to the United States.

In contrast, two European studies found that countries with different degrees of welfare state provisions nevertheless had similar patterns of health inequities: one investigation compared 11 European countries on four measures of morbidity and observed that the Nordic countries did not have less relative education-based health inequality than the remaining non-social democratic states, while another reported that magnitude of health inequities in two subjective measures for single compared to married mothers was similar in Finland and Britain despite their different policy provisions for single mothers. Additionally, three studies reported increases in health inequities following expansion of the welfare state: in Spain, in Finland, and in Norway. The point is that the effect of the welfare state on health in rich democracies is very much up for grabs and would benefit from engagement by political sociologists. In such engagement, it will be crucial to maintain the social-epidemiological distinction between relative and absolute differences.

In a recent contribution to this debate, the Health Inequalities in European Welfare States (HiNEWS) project reported new analyses of European Social Survey (ESS) data, which incorporated a new health module in its 2014 wave. The HiNEWS team published 16 papers in a recent supplement to the *European Journal of Public Health*. In many cases, the most surprising result, from the perspective of mainstream biomedical, behavioral, psychosocial, and materialist perspectives, is that the "usual suspects" of individual-level biological factors and health behaviors contribute fairly little to the explanation of health and healthcare inequities. While this is an important challenge to the dominant approaches to disease distribution and healthcare utilization, it is not affirmative evidence of the importance of institutional arrangements in welfare states. It is, instead, an invitation to further analysis of how such factors might matter for health and healthcare inequities above and beyond the usual individual biological and behavioral factors.

The first surprising theme across several articles is the documentation of cross-national variability in the magnitude and patterning of health inequity. For instance, one survey of self-reported conditions shows that chronic conditions are prevalent in European populations, at rates that vary from 45% of the population to 92% of the population, even after age adjustment. Moreover, gender differences in the experience of chronic conditions are themselves highly variable across national context, lending *prima facie* support to the "constrained choices" approach developed by Bird and Rieker (2008) to explain cross-national variation in gender-based health inequity. Another article shifts from gender to geography and reveals high heterogeneity in the distribution of chronic illness across places in Europe. A key result from this paper goes against the "Nordic Paradox" of large relative inequalities in mortality rates in universalistic welfare states, finding instead the lowest levels of absolute and relative inequalities in chronic illness in Denmark, Norway, and Sweden. As important, the extent of place-based inequity itself varies substantially across European nations and is especially large in Germany, a federation of states with substantial autonomy in the design of social and healthcare policy.

The second surprising theme across articles is the cross-national variability in the extent to which health behaviors, sometimes assumed to have constant and universal health "outputs" for the same "inputs," vary across populations in their contribution to health inequity. One study demonstrates that, although there are strong relationships between health behaviors and measures of physical and mental health in representative samples of several European nations, the patterns of exposure to these behavioral risks vary substantially cross-nationally, as do their effects. This article thus casts doubt on the argument that the "health penalty" of an unhealthy behavior like smoking is a biological constant, and instead shows how such penalties are institutionally patterned (for more on cross-national variation in "prevalences and penalties," see Brady, Finnigan, & Hübgen, 2017). Thus, the mediating role of health behaviors in translating socioeconomic status inequality into health inequity is a structural variable, not a biological constant. A second article examines the extent to which engagement in risky behavior—measured as excessive alcohol consumption, smoking, and avoiding fruits and vegetables—explains why better-educated people experience less chronic illness than less-educated people. Once again the results cast doubt on the argument that risky health behavior is a constant and universal mediator between socioeconomic status inequality and health inequity. Instead, the results show substantial cross-national variation in not only the prevalence of risky behavior, but also the health effects of risky behavior, which may be connected to cross-national differences in political variables such as taxation and healthcare systems.

The third surprising theme is that the *effects* of chronic illness are distributed unevenly across social groups, and those inequities themselves are unevenly distributed across national populations. One article documents this cross-national variation using the experience of cancer as a case. The key insight is that even an illness as serious as cancer varies strongly in its effects on quality of life, with people in some countries suffering much worse than others. Notably, the broad, three-category welfare-state classification does not seem to explain the cross-national variation that exists in the extent to which cancer undermines quality of life. Several of the articles highlighted in the preceding sections also support a "variable-penalty" approach to chronic illness, since the cross-sectional data in the ESS do not allow for a rigorous assessment of causal direction.

The U.S. Mortality Disadvantage

While investigations of European welfare states and European health inequalities continue to produce evidence for and against the basic hypothesis that welfare states enhance health equality, the evidence is somewhat clearer that between-country differences in welfare states contribute to between-country differences in population health.

One striking dimension of the global distribution of health is the U.S. mortality and morbidity disadvantage. In 1960, Scandinavian nations topped the life-expectancy-at-birth list of 18 high-income OECD (Organization for Economic Cooperation and Development) nations, with Norway's life expectancy of 73.8 years (OECD, 2012). The United States ranked 15th, with a life expectancy of 69.8 years. The average life expectancy at birth for the 18 OECD countries in 1960 was 70.8 years. By 2010, the United States had dropped to the bottom of the relative rankings, with a life expectancy of 78.7 years compared to 83.0 years in table-topping Japan (OECD, 2012). The average in 2010 was 81.0 years. Mortality in the United States changed over this period to such an extent that the gap between the highest life expectancy and the United States' life expectancy grew from 4.0 years in 1960 to 4.3 years in 2010. Again based on OECD Health Data, the pattern is actually worse for the infant mortality rate. In 1960, four of the six nations with the lowest infant mortality rates were Scandinavian, and the United States ranked 11th, with an infant mortality rate of 26.0, double Iceland's rate of 13.0. By 2010, this relative difference grew. Scandinavian nations still dominated the top ranks, while the United States dropped to the bottom of the list with an infant mortality rate of 6.1—nearly triple table-topping Iceland's rate of 2.2 and almost double the average of 3.7.

This U.S. health disadvantage was the subject of a recent report by the U.S. National Academies: *Shorter Lives, Poorer Health: U.S. Health in International Perspective* (Woolf & Aron, 2013). It found that currently the United States does worse than comparator rich democratic countries across at least nine health domains:

1. adverse birth outcomes—the United States has the worst infant mortality rates, worst rates of low birthweight babies, and U.S. children are less likely to live to age five than children in other high-income countries;
2. injuries and homicide—deaths from motor vehicle crashes, injuries, and violence occur at a much higher rate than in other countries;
3. the United States has the highest rate of teenage pregnancies and young people are more likely to acquire sexually transmitted diseases;
4. the United States has the highest incidence of AIDS;
5. U.S. adults lost more years of life to alcohol or drugs;
6. U.S. obesity and diabetes rates are the highest in the world for those aged over 20 years;
7. U.S. adults aged over 50 are more likely to die from heart disease than those in other countries;
8. lung disease is more common in the United States; and
9. disability rates are higher than most other high-income nations.

These issues are universal across the social/spatial gradient— with the poorest areas and social groups faring worse than the poorest areas or social groups of other countries, and more affluent areas and social groups faring worse than their status peers in other countries.

The poor recent health performance of the United States relative to other rich democracies began in the 1980s (Woolf & Aron, 2013). Recently, scholars have begun to identify the potential political roots of this change, building on the robust result that cross-national inequality in mortality rates started growing first among U.S. women who experienced premature mortality and higher rates of mortality at older ages. This cohort of women was the generation that included the mothers of the baby-boomers; that is, women who were themselves born in the 1910s–1930s (recall that the fertility rate during the Baby Boom peaked in 1960 in the U.S.). These women were among the first to enter the paid labor market in large numbers, and thus, combined with high fertility rates, were among the first to experience lifecourse histories of strong work–family conflict (Sabbath, Guevara, Glymour, & Berkman, 2015).

Building on the insight that social policies have the capacity to support women and families, and thus might play a role in the development of this added mortality burden among older women in the United States, research using newly available life-history data from the U.S. Health and Retirement Study and the European Survey of Health, Aging, and Retirement has shown that U.S. women followed work–family trajectories similar to those of their European peers (van Hedel et al., 2016). This suggests that the different welfare-state contexts may have changed the experience of work–family combinations for women in these age cohorts. Consistent with this scenario is evidence that more generous maternity leave policies improve maternal mental health over the lifecourse in Europe (Avendano, Berkman, Brugiavini, & Pasini, 2015).

How much do these social policy differences contribute to the U.S. health disadvantage? Research on welfare-state effects on health inequalities is developing rapidly. One recent study suggests that life expectancy in the United States would be as much as 3.77 years longer if the United States had an even average level of social policy generosity. If the United States had the high level of universal benefits provided in Nordic welfare states, U.S. life expectancy would be as much as 5.56 years longer, based on these estimates. Table 2.2 reports the estimates, which come from a regression decomposition that compares the United States to two counterfactual scenarios: an average OECD welfare state, and an average Nordic welfare state.

Income Inequality and Health Inequality

While the relationship between the welfare state and *health inequality* is uncertain, especially in European welfare states, there is little doubt that welfare states are closely associated with *income inequality*. There is an ongoing, heated debate among comparative health researchers over whether the level of income inequality in a society is associated with aggregate, societal-level measures of population health such as the infant mortality rate and life expectancy (Beckfield, 2004; Jen et al., 2009; Kim et al., 2008; Wilkinson & Pickett, 2006). That is, there is dissensus on the existence of a relationship between inequality and health. Zimmerman (2008) provocatively notes that research on the association between inequality and health is now generating "far more heat than light, with two dug-in

Table 2.2 Decomposition of the U.S. Life Expectancy Disadvantage Suggests Americans Would Live Several Years Longer if the United States Were Not a Welfare Laggard

Regression Decomposition of the U.S. Life Expectancy Disadvantage
U.S. vs. 17 OECD Nations

	U.S.	OECD
b_{Year} (s.e.)	0.149	0.221
	(0.005)	(0.004)
$b_{Generosity}$ (s.e.)	0.311	0.006
	(0.050)	(0.007)
Constant (s.e.)	65.7	71.9
	(0.987)	(0.231)

Endowments effect (change in U.S. LE if U.S. had OECD-average generosity): 3.77 (s.e. = 0.657)

Coefficients effect (change in U.S. LE if U.S. had OECD coefficients): 1.29 (s.e. = 0.146)

Interaction between endowments effect and coefficients effect: −3.38 (s.e. = 0.590)

U.S. vs. Nordic Nations (Denmark, Finland, Norway, and Sweden)

	U.S.	Nordic
b_{Year} (s.e.)	0.149	0.168
	(0.005)	(0.006)
$b_{Generosity}$ (s.e.)	0.311	0.154
	(0.050)	(0.016)
Constant (s.e.)	65.7	67.4
	(0.987)	(0.231)

Endowments effect (change in U.S. LE if U.S. had Nordic-average generosity): 5.56 (s.e. = 0.950)

Coefficients effect (change in U.S. LE if U.S. had Nordic coefficients): −1.24 (s.e. = 0.302)

Interaction between endowments effect and coefficients effect: −2.74 (s.e. = 0.928)

Note: b is a regression coefficient estimate, s.e. is a standard error, and OECD is the Organization for Economic Cooperation and Development. Please see Beckfield and Bambra (2016) for methodological details.

sides lobbing analyses back and forth with increasing sophistication and decreasing effect" (Zimmerman, 2008, p. 1882). One way to generate some light is to examine whether and to what degree economic inequality in a society—as measured across a population, as well as spatially within a population—influences inequalities in health.

Why should economic inequality be positively associated with the level of inequality in health? Imagine that the effect of individual income on individual health is the same in two societies, but one has higher levels of income inequality, making the association between income and health stronger, mechanically, in the higher-income-inequality society. In addition, individuals with either educational or income advantage in a higher-income-inequality society may have even more resources that they can translate even more effectively into better health, and the poor would be even more deeply disadvantaged (Evans, Hout, & Meyer, 2004; Hout & Fisher, 2003). Furthermore, if income serves as a buffer against the strains of everyday life (Hall & Lamont, 2009), lower-income people in higher-inequality societies should be less healthy, generating a steeper gradient. Finally, if income inequality is an accurate index of the general level of social inequality in a society (in other words, if income inequality captures social stratification in a very general way), then income inequality should be positively associated with measures of health inequality.

Evidence on the educational gradient in all-cause mortality shows that the U.S. mortality disadvantage results in part from the greater "penalty" of low educational attainment in the United States relative to Belgium, Denmark, Finland, France, Norway, Sweden, and Switzerland (van Hedel et al., 2015). The reasons for this are still unclear, but it could be that the high level of general social inequality in the United States makes individual resources—private goods—like the human capital of educational attainment more important in securing health. Figure 2.12 shows evidence on

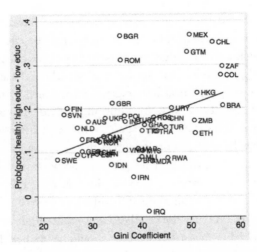

Figure 2.12 *In countries with more income inequality, the education gradient in self-rated health is steeper.*

Source: Beckfield et al, American Behavioral Scientist, 2013. Countries shown are Australia (AUS), Burkina Faso (BFA), Bulgaria (BGR), Brazil (BRA), Canada (CAN), Chile (CHL), China (CHN), Columbia (COL), Cyprus (CYP), Ethiopia (ETH), Finland (FIN), France (FRA), Great Britain (GBR), Germany (GER), Ghana (GHA), Guatemala (GTM), Hong Kong (HKG), India (IND), Indonesia (IDN), Iran (IRN), Iraq (IRQ), Italy (ITA), Japan (JPN), Morocco (MAR), Moldova (MDA), Mexico (MEX), Mali (MLI), Malaysia (MYS), Netherlands (NLD), Poland (POL), Romania (ROM), Russia (RUS), Rwanda (RWA), Slovenia (SVN), South Africa (ZAF), South Korea (KOR), Spain (ESP), Sweden (SWE), Switzerland (CHE), Thailand (THA), Trinidad and Tobago (TTO), Turkey (TUR), Taiwan (TWN), Ukraine (UKR), Uruguay (URY), United States (USA), Vietnam (VNM), and Zambia (ZMB).

that relationship from a different study, which compared health inequalities in a wide variety of countries with data available from the World Values Study (Beckfield et al., 2013).

In the figure, the data points represent the difference in predicted probabilities of reporting good health, for people with relatively high vs. relatively low levels of educational attainment, from country-specific logistic regression models that also include age, sex, income, and marital status. These differences in predicted probabilities are shown by the level of income inequality in each country, where income inequality is measured as the Gini coefficient. The figure shows that income inequality does seem to be associated with the steepness of the education gradient in health: more unequal societies are also places where the private good of educational attainment matters more for one's own health.

Political Economy: Neoliberalism, Austerity, Capitalism, and Collective Bargaining

As discussed in the last chapter, the political economy concept captures multiple institutional arrangements that structure relations between states and markets. Relatively few have been examined for their impact on the distribution of population health, but exceptions are studies of neoliberal reforms and austerity policies; the transition to capitalism in former Communist countries; and labor unions as collective bargaining institutions that organize power relations between employers and employees.

Eight studies reviewed by Krieger and I (Beckfield & Krieger, 2009) tested hypotheses regarding the impact of neoliberal political and economic reforms of the 1980s and 1990s on health inequities. Four focused on mortality—and three found that neoliberal reforms were associated with increased health inequities, including two New Zealand studies on education- and income-based relative disparities in adult mortality rates and child mortality, and a U.S. study on relative and absolute income and racial/ethnic inequities in premature mortality and infant mortality. By contrast, one study found that, at least for premature mortality, relative health inequity in New Zealand during its period of neoliberal reform did not increase more than it did in Denmark, Finland, and Norway, where there were less intensive neoliberal reforms. Among the four studies focused on non-mortality health outcomes, one in New Zealand found evidence of post-neoliberal reform increases in Maori–European relative and absolute inequality in the dental caries experience of children, whereas the three studies with self-rated health as the outcome (all Scandinavian) found stable education- and gender-based relative and absolute inequalities during the period of neoliberal reforms in Sweden, Norway, and Finland.

While neoliberal reforms marked macroscopic political and economic change in Europe and New Zealand in the 1980s and 1990s, former Communist countries experienced even more dramatic changes as they transitioned to market economies. Many experienced rapid out-migration, especially among younger people, and dramatic increases in mortality, especially from alcohol- and smoking-related causes of death. In this context, nine studies test the hypothesis that (class-based) health inequities grow in the period immediately following the transition to capitalism, and eight found supportive evidence in terms of growing relative or absolute education-related health inequities. Outcomes included: for Russia, overall and cause-specific mortality, with one study finding evidence against the hypothesis that this was driven by growing inequality in alcohol consumption; and, for Poland, East Germany, Estonia, the Czech Republic, and Lithuania, premature mortality, unhealthy housing conditions for children, life expectancy, birthweight and preterm delivery, and all-cause mortality. The one negative study focused on self-rated health in Estonia, Latvia, and Lithuania, with Finland serving as a control.

Reynolds and Brady (2012) provide one of the only studies to document a robust association between union membership and health, in this case, self-rated health as measured in the U.S. General Social Survey between 1973 and 2006. Acknowledging and testing for selection effects driven by unmeasured differences between union members and non-union members, Reynolds and Brady argue that union membership enhances self-rated health through direct and indirect channels. Direct channels include workplace safety and health protections, long a priority of labor unions, and social determinants of health such as higher incomes. Indirect channels include power resources, as labor unions enhance the power of workers relative to employers. Their evidence shows statistically significant effects of labor union membership on health, including an average treatment effect on the treated from a propensity score matching analysis. The size of the effect of labor union membership is substantial, and comparable to the effect of five years of aging, or the difference between married and divorced people. This suggests union decline in the United States as another candidate explanation for the U.S. mortality disadvantage.

3 | SCIENTIFIC CHALLENGES TO ENGAGING POLITICAL SOCIOLOGY AND SOCIAL EPIDEMIOLOGY

As detailed in Chapter 1, political sociology offers a rich array of concepts and measures for investigating how institutional arrangements contribute to the distribution of population health. As Chapter 2 described, only some of these concepts and measures have been considered in social-epidemiological research, despite the ongoing turn toward upstream variables that put people "at risk of risks" for diseases and death. That is, social epidemiology demonstrates clearly that social structure has profound consequences for the distribution of health, illness, and death, but it remains the case that political-sociological variables tend to be imprecisely incorporated into social epidemiological models. If the preceding chapters suggest how researchers could make a start on such incorporation, this chapter highlights the challenges to doing so in a convincing manner. Table 3.1 summarizes these challenges.

Explaining Embodiment

The concept of embodiment evokes a general set of processes whereby people incorporate the multiple ecologies we live in,

Table 3.1 Challenges to Engagement Between Political Sociology and Social Epidemiology

Challenge	Summary	Example	Further Reading
Explaining Embodiment	Explanation requires new theory, data, and analysis of synchronous, asynchronous, cumulative, and heterogeneous causation	Political-sociological exposures are embodied across the lifecourse; e.g., Jim Crow and premature mortality, and maternity leave and women's mental health	Avendano et al., 2015; Beckfield et al., 2015; Krieger, 2011; Krieger et al., 2014; Xie, 2013
Combining Epistemologies	Epidemiology relies on quantification, but political sociology is pluralistic	New approaches offer systematic ways to integrate qualitative and quantitative evidence	Lieberman, 2005; Small, 2011
Establishing Causation	Counterfactual causation risks narrowing types of causes considered	Fundamental causes, necessary but insufficient causes, and sufficient but not necessary causes may require special identification strategies	Freese & Kevern, 2013; Lieberson, 1985
Observing Mechanisms	Processes that link political sociological causes to social epidemiological effects (and vice versa) should be theorized, but may not always be measurable within a single study design	A pluralistic approach to integrating evidence within and across studies can help identify mechanisms; e.g., through a process of elimination	Hedström & Bearman, 2009; Killewald & Gough, 2013; Liu, King, & Bearman, 2010

Creating Comparability	Unmeasured heterogeneity among cases arguably matters more when Ns are small, and there are tradeoffs between large-N and small-N macro-comparisons	Comparability of people is widely accepted despite unmeasured heterogeneity, but not so with populations; repeated measures allow for estimation of fixed- or random-effects models; case studies are required for identification of temporal processes	Davidov, Meuleman, Cieciuch, Schmidt, & Billiet, 2014; Ebbinghaus, 2005; Halaby, 2004; Lieberson, 1991
Theorizing Timing	Political-sociological exposures and embodiment unfold over time, so a pressing theoretical challenge is to conceptualize historical processes, feedback effects, and path dependencies	The power of households to produce health among their members was central to long-run mortality reductions, in ways that shaped the evolution of causes of death differently by etiologic period	Clemens, 2007; Krieger, Singh, et al., 2015; Pierson, 2004; Riley, 2001

(continued)

Table 3.1 Continued

Challenge	Summary	Example	Further Reading
Measuring Dependencies	People and polities are interdependent in complex social, historical, and spatial ways, but dominant statistical methods often assume independence of units	Network relations among people are measured in such resources as the National Longitudinal Study of Adolescent Health; and among polities in such resources as the Correlates of War data; migration data from the Mexican Migration Project and the Nang Rong Surveys include network, migration, health, and political-sociological measures	Bearman, Moody, & Stovel, 2004; Curran, Garip, Chung, & Tangchonlatip, 2005; DiMaggio & Garip, 2012; Garip, 2008; Pevehouse, Nordstrom, & Warnke, 2004
Placing Inequalities	Connections among political sociological exposures, the distribution of population health, and spatial ecology are under-theorized	Exceptions are research on racial, residential, and occupational sex segregation; new research that uses the Index of Concentration at the Extremes to estimate neighborhood socio-political ecological effects; and emerging work on climate change and health inequities	Feldman, Waterman, Coull, & Krieger, 2015; Krieger, Waterman, Gryparis, & Coull, 2015; Massey & Denton, 1993; Noelke et al., 2016; Pettit & Hook, 2009; Sampson, 2012

simultaneously and over the life course. This generality, multiplicity, and simultaneity challenge the development of convincing explanations, because these processes can seem to include everything and locate themselves everywhere and nowhere. If the challenge is to explain how, when, why, and for whom embodiment happens, one approach to explanation is to consider the abstract properties of the body itself as an *explanandum*. Unlike the outcomes typically explained by political sociologists interested in social inequality, which include employment, wages, poverty, and income inequality, the materiality of the body and its development over time mean that in explaining embodiment, we are explaining something with a potentially different causal structure. These differences are summarized in Table 3.2.

Consider, for example, the difference between income inequality, which is investigated as an outcome by many political sociologists, and health inequality, which is arguably the core *explanandum* of social epidemiology. Income inequality is simply the

Table 3.2 **Comparison of the Etiology (Causal Structure) of Income, Wealth, and Death**

Outcome	Dimensions	Timing	Origin
Income	Market, State	Simultaneous	Organizations
Wealth	Assets, Debt, Financial Assets	Cumulative	Family, Career
Death	Age-Specific, Cause-Specific, Cohort-Specific	Simultaneous, Cumulative, Asynchronous	Age-Specific, Cause-Specific, Cohort-Specific

quantity of dispersion in incomes, usually measured at the household or individual level. Of course, many measures are available, but they all rely on individual- or household-level income for their calculation. And so how should we conceptualize the etiology—the general causal structure—of income? People can earn income from many sources, including markets (labor, housing, and finance among them) and states (pensions, health care, and unemployment among them). To develop a cross-nationally comparable data resource for the investigation of income inequality, the Luxembourg Income Study developed an income concept that synthesized decades of work from multiple fields, and heterogeneous structural realities across dozens of countries. And yet, the dimensionality of income is much narrower than that of the many aspects of health, illness, and mortality that describe embodiment. Dozens if not hundreds of elaborately validated and statistically reliable measures describe mental health and physical health, and thousands of mental and physical health disorders have been identified. For instance, the International Standard Classification of Disease, which many countries use to identify diagnoses and causes of death, includes over 16,000 codes.

This radical difference in dimensionality is joined with striking differences between income and health in etiological timing and relations. That is, their causal structures differ in the social relations involved, and in the role of time in causal processes. The timing of income is synchronous: very generally, most wage laborers are paid for labor completed over the near-term past. Again very generally, income from public sources comes from current or near-term past conditions (current health conditions that require sick pay or disability pay, current unemployment status, current retirement status). In contrast, many diseases—including some of the major causes of death—only develop over a longer time scale. Heart disease, for instance, develops after the accumulation of long-term bodily insults from accumulated allostatic load and inflammation. Lung disease, one of the top five causes of death in rich democracies, also tends to develop over decades. So, too, with AIDS-related diseases, which are top causes of death in several low-income countries. In contrast, other illnesses and causes of death have much shorter etiologic periods; these include infectious diseases like malaria, viral infections like influenza, and accidents like vehicular and firearm deaths.

The social relations in the etiology of health also differ from those in the etiology of income. In the case of income, family, employment, and citizenship relations constitute the majority of the social relations that cause variation in income. In the case of well-being, illness, and mortality, the set of directly causal social relations is much broader, and includes the experience of interactional discrimination, gendered interaction, social dominance, collective efficacy in neighborhoods, social support, social isolation, health care, and many others. To be clear, it is not that the larger set of social relations does not affect income, but those effects of income are channeled through organized family, employment, and citizenship relations. The etiology of health includes these relationships in a much broader complex of relations.

For political sociologists newly engaging social epidemiology, one approach to developing hypotheses about the factors that explain embodiment is to start with the body. Mainstream risk-factor organ-centered epidemiology has established facts about the etiology of many diseases and causes of death, and such knowledge can be used to develop hypotheses about political-sociological explanations for health inequalities that result from embodiment processes. For example, infant mortality has a short-term etiological structure that responds quickly to deprivation above and beyond the important role of the mother's preconception health. Therefore, political-sociological changes that alter the distribution of deprivation in the short term should affect inequality in infant mortality. This is the approach taken in a study of the effect of dismantling Jim Crow in the United States via the Civil Rights Acts of 1964 and 1965 on racial inequality in infant mortality. By comparing blacks living in Jim Crow states to blacks living in non–Jim-Crow states—to identify the causal effect of living different institutional arrangements—the study was able to show a strong effect of political incorporation on reducing infant mortality caused by broad-scale, racialized, political, social, and economic deprivation (Krieger et al., 2013).

Timing is just one element of the etiological complexity of health, illness, and death. The social relations and dimensionality of etiology must also be considered in the development of hypotheses that can contribute to the explanation of embodiment. Candidate political-sociological causes of health inequalities can be identified by joining the social epidemiology of specific measures of health, illness, and disease with a general framework of institutional causation. Recall that the political-sociological concept "institution" is an umbrella term that captures the schemas and resources involved in establishing and enforcing the rules of the game that guide social and political life. In hypothesis-building to explain embodiment, substantive knowledge from social epidemiology can be combined with a general institutional framework for the explanation of health inequalities. Such a framework can then guide the research collaboration, by identifying the area of substantive political-sociological knowledge required to generate specific hypotheses and identify state-of-the-art measures.

At the level of general theory, the argument of this book is that political-sociological structures and processes affect inequality in the distribution of social goods (health, income, wealth, poverty) through direct redistribution (in the case of welfare-state income transfers) and predistribution; constraints on the distribution of outcomes (in the case of a minimum wage); through other determinants (in the case of incarceration, which raises the probability of exclusion from paid employment in the U.S.); and by influencing selection processes. For political sociologists, a benefit of engaging with social epidemiology is to broaden the array of stratified goods that are distributed by institutions, including the many elements of socioeconomic position. That is, this developing institutional theory holds that inequality in some variable Y can be explained in part by institutional factors that

1. shift Y from people who have more Y to people who have less Y (or vice versa, through regressive taxation),
2. limit how low or high Y can go for different population groups,
3. affect other variables such as X that themselves affect Y and its distribution,
4. combine multiple policy exposures and channel their overlapping effects to variable parts of the population, and
5. differentially select individuals into the causes of health effects (Beckfield et al., 2015).

These can be conceptualized as modifications to the quincunx discussed previously. For social epidemiologists, a benefit of engaging with this political-sociological approach to institutions is that novel explanations of embodiment can be identified. This approach is summarized in Table 3.3, which also provides examples of the schemas and resources involved in each institutional mechanism, describes the kind of power being organized in each case, and gives examples of political-sociological institutions that may be relevant to social inequalities in health.

I argue that these institutional mechanisms are helpful in thinking not only about the distribution of health, but also about the distribution of the social determinants of health (Osypuk et al., 2014). These five institutional mechanisms—redistribution, compression, mediation, imbrication, and selection—identify how the institutional factors that might help to explain embodiment can be developed. Consider the example of how welfare states contribute to embodiment. In European welfare states, the reason social inequalities in health are surprising is that health care has long been considered and delivered as a citizenship right, as have other areas of social provision such as income support for the unemployed. At least for citizens, then (the picture is more complicated if we include non-citizen migrants), the redistribution (e.g., income redistribution as an institutional effect on one of the social determinants of health), compression, and mediation channels from institutions to inequality should be working to reduce health inequality. That is, welfare states set a minimum bound for the healthcare of citizens (compression, which happens in part as regulations of healthcare access), and they limit inequality in some of the factors that have been established as robust

Table 3.3 Summary of the Institutional Theory of Social Inequalities in Health

Mechanism	X and Y	Schema	Resources	Power	Example
Redistribution	Shift X (social goods) from/ to people with more/less X	In/egalitarianism	Fiscal policy	Control over social goods	Regressive taxation policy
Compression	Limit the minimum or maximum Y (floors/ ceilings)	Moral logic of un/acceptability	Public health care, medical technology	Market interaction	Neonatal intensive care units
Mediation	Strengthen or weaken the effect of X on Y by affecting X	Unanticipated mechanical effect	Multiple	Strategy: toolkit composition	Educational expansion that shifts the distribution of attainment
Imbrication (Overlapping Institutions)	Combine political exposures and channel them to population	Safety net, exposure to social risks	Eligibility and public/private provision	Market interaction	Welfare regime (conservative, liberal, social democratic)
Selection	Distribution of low/high X to part of population through organizational processes	Universalistic/ particularistic	Organizational, legal	Social reproduction and boundaries	Educational attainment and social (im)mobility

social determinants of health, such as income (mediation). States also shape the importance of selection into health-consequential conditions like unemployment.

From a political-sociological perspective, the complexity of population health distribution in an institutional context represents an invitation to theoretical development. Any measure of health inequality is a snapshot, taken at one moment in the evolution of a population, that compares the health of one socially defined category of people to another. For instance, women aged 45–64 with a university degree could be compared to same-aged women with a lower level of educational attainment than a university degree, on the common metric of a depression scale, blood pressure, or mortality risk over a defined period. An institutional theory explains this health inequality as a function of redistribution (shifting social determinants of health like income and wealth), compression (institutional arrangements that provide health care directly, thereby lowering rates of the most common illnesses for this group), mediation (institutional arrangements that reduce educational inequality), imbrication (the overlap among safety-net policies across different age groups and other politically defined populations), and selection (policies that make it more or less likely that this category of people will have been selected from some social origins over others). These effects can be reinforcing, but they can also be cross-cutting.

This example illustrates well the theoretical complexity in understanding how health inequalities respond to institutions. Illnesses vary greatly in etiologic period, with some like heart disease emerging over decades, and others like anxiety attacks emerging quickly (albeit sometimes chronically) in response to disruption. Populations evolve over time, as people are born, migrate, and die. People carry with them early-life conditions, such that an educational system in early adulthood determines educational inequality throughout the lifecourse. At the same time, institutions change, sometimes slower than bodies, but sometimes faster. People within a population at any one time may therefore have experiences with different welfare state lifecourses (Bambra, Netuveli, & Eikemo, 2010). Insights from the extensive literature on the lifecourse should be synthesized with social epidemiological knowledge about disease etiology, and comparative-historical evidence on institutional change (Hall & Taylor, 1996; Korpi & Palme, 1998).

Another theoretical challenge that arises in the case of health inequality—in part because welfare state institutions have direct and indirect effects on health—is the potential of cross-cutting or amplifying institutional effects across institutional domains. That is, welfare states can stratify health through health care, and, simultaneously, through the distribution of other valued goods that themselves operate as social determinants of health (such as employment security and precarity). With respect to inequalities in mortality, the institutional effect of healthcare institutions may be restricted to amenable mortality, while other welfare state institutions through their impact on social determinants of health also create inequalities in mortality that are not directly affected by the healthcare system (Newey, Nolte, McKee, & Mossialos, 2003). I conceptualize this simultaneous operation of institutions in multiple domains at multiple levels as institutional imbrication (where the concept of imbrication draws on Sassen's work; see Sassen, 2006). Institutional imbrication is the overlapping of two or more institutions, such as when the educational system distributes resources that are themselves important within the healthcare system. For instance, a highly stratified educational system would amplify health inequality in situations where complex treatment regimes produce strong educational gradients in health care. Imbrication allows for amplifying, cross-cutting, or moderating effects of institutional arrangements, accurately reflecting the reality that people "live" more than one policy at a time over the life course.

Note that this perspective would take into account the role of multiple disadvantages to explain the persistence of social inequalities in health in welfare states. By mostly targeting the financial dimension of disadvantage, welfare states may have neglected the fact that financial adversity is often paralleled by other dimensions of disadvantage. People who are most in need of financial compensation by the welfare state also have lower educational levels, less social support, and smaller social networks. Additionally, financial disadvantage is found more among social groups that face discrimination and social exclusion, such as women (especially lone mothers) and ethnic minorities (Bryant & Raphael, 2005). This connects to Sen's capability approach, a general framework holding that people will only be able to translate endowments (such as sufficient financial means) into capabilities (such as the ability to pursue a healthy life) if they possess sufficient "conversion factors" (e.g., cognitive or social resources that are themselves distributed by institutional arrangements). Based on this general framework, people may only be able to turn the financial compensation and other incentives provided by the welfare state into health benefits if they have the right resources (private household, or public welfare) at their disposal to do so (Bartley, 2003).

Such resources are located at multiple levels of analysis. For example, at the individual level, people will benefit more from welfare arrangements if their educational level is higher (e.g., because of better knowledge on how to make adequate use of healthcare services provided by the welfare state). At the macro level, social norms may facilitate the use of welfare arrangements by disadvantaged groups (e.g., in societies with norms that are positive toward working women, lone mothers will be more prone to use subsidized child care arrangements offered by the welfare state). Turning to the institutional level, specific institutional arrangements determine whether welfare beneficiaries can use their higher educational status for choosing child care, health care, or other welfare arrangements, or not (Reibling & Wendt, 2012, 2013).

Note also that the institutional arrangements that distribute population health through redistribution, compression, mediation, imbrication, and selection need not be exclusively or even mostly national in scope. That is, arrangements that blur the boundaries of welfare should be incorporated in the endeavor to build a theory of the distribution of population health that takes globalization (and other forms of transnational interaction, such as regional integration) seriously by problematizing the very boundaries of institutions (Ferrera, 2005).

Epistemology

While the field of social epidemiology tilts very heavily toward quantitative analysis, political sociology is much more evenly balanced, with major headway on the reproduction of social inequality, the exercise of power, and the processes of social exclusion made by ethnographic and interview–based research. Likewise, both qualitative and quantitative studies have advanced the political sociology of institutions and welfare states. Currently, many sociologists and political scientists are working on the systematic integration of qualitative and quantitative research as a general epistemological matter (Lieberman, 2005; Small, 2011). Still, because of the strong quantitative bias of epidemiological research, method poses a big challenge to engagement between political sociology and social epidemiology. For instance, qualitative, in-depth interviews and close observation of a small number of people in social settings might not be considered "data" by some epidemiologists, a view that is more nuanced in social branches of epidemiology.

Causation

The dominant framework for the evaluation of causation in social epidemiology is currently the counterfactual approach, which rests on the logic of experimental manipulation. This approach is discussed and debated in a recent exchange published by the *International Journal of Epidemiology* (Blakely, Lynch, & Bentley, 2016; Krieger & Davey Smith, 2016; Robins & Weissman, 2016; Vandenbroucke, Broadbent, & Pearce, 2016; VanderWeele, Hernán, Tchetgen Tchetgen, & Robins, 2016; Weed, 2016). Unfortunately, this focus on the counterfactual approach to causation has led to the neglect of other varieties of causation. These include fundamental causes that represent systems of relations among regular causes (e.g., socioeconomic position causes health and illness via "massively multiple mechanisms" [Lutfey

& Freese 2005]), necessary but insufficient conditions (e.g., component causes), and sufficient but unnecessary conditions (e.g., precipitating causes) (Freese & Kevern, 2013). Arguably, political-sociological exposures are especially likely to be fundamental, component, and precipitating causes, which are difficult to study within the confines of counterfactual causal logics (Brady, Blome, et al., 2016).

Mechanisms

Social epidemiology and political sociology share a growing concern with identifying and measuring the mechanisms (or processes) that connect causes to effects. This has been a major challenge to the integration of political sociology and social epidemiology, since few datasets exist that combine macroscopic institutional exposures and individual health outcomes over longer periods of time. Thus, a striking characteristic of extant research in this area is that causal mechanisms are rarely tested directly. Of the 45 studies Beckfield and Krieger reviewed, only six actually investigated mechanisms. Of course, it is not always possible within the confines of a single study to identify and measure all the processes that connect cause to effect, and exemplary studies make important scientific progress through processes of elimination (Killewald & Gough, 2013; Liu et al., 2010).

Typically, in studies relating political-sociological exposures to health inequities, if mechanisms are addressed at all, appeal is made to secondary research on hierarchy stress (the argument being that institutions that flatten hierarchies reduce stress and elevate health, presumably by reducing cardiovascular disease). Rarely, arguments are made that connect specific social policies to specific groups that benefit from those policies; for example, Olafsdottir used survey data from Iceland and the United States to show that parents are healthier in Iceland than in the United States, at least in part because of the more generous family policy of the Icelandic welfare state (Olafsdottir, 2007). It remains to be seen how institutional interaction—how people engage with institutions—may represent a key mechanism for welfare state effects on health inequalities, though U.S. evidence is suggestive (Gage-Bouchard, 2017). One macro-level study of political-sociological exposures and population health that attends closely to potential (unobserved) mechanisms is by Conley and Springer, who disaggregate different kinds of infant mortality to bolster the inference that the welfare state (through investments in health technology) reduces infant mortality more strongly in more generous welfare states (Conley & Springer, 2001). Unfortunately, though, fixed-effects models are blunt tools that cannot estimate effects of *longue-durée* changes.

Comparability

In order to evaluate embodied social inequalities in different settings, the comparability of the data is of course essential. This means that variables should be measured consistently across cases, a substantial challenge when measuring health inequities across societies with different legal systems, languages, cultures, and social structures (Davidov et al., 2014). One setting where significant progress has been made on comparability is in comparative healthcare systems research. Currently, there is a wealth of cross-nationally comparable data on healthcare arrangements and national institutions available to researchers. These data can largely be divided into two types: data that address the scope and the nature of the healthcare system itself, and data that evaluate public opinion about the healthcare system. Also, the anchoring-vignette method has now been used in many cross-national studies to improve comparability, or at least the assessment of comparability.

Both the Organization for Economic Cooperation and Development (OECD) and the World Health Organization (WHO) offer data on comparative healthcare systems, with the former limited to the 30 OECD countries (mostly advanced, industrialized nations), and the latter offering a larger sample of nations. These data include spending on health care, the proportion of the population with access to health care, the number of certain medical procedures performed annually, and the number of medical doctors per a given population. Some research has used this kind of data to evaluate differences in healthcare systems, offering different typologies for healthcare systems (Wendt, Frisina, & Rothgang, 2009; Wendt, Grimmeisen, & Rothgang, 2005). The next step in such research could be to show how the differences in the organization of healthcare systems impact healthcare disparities and health disparities.

Several cross-national studies offer insights into how the public feels about the healthcare system and how it is working. For example, the International Social Survey Programme (ISSP) offers questions on the role of the government in health care, and the European Social Survey (ESS) has included rotating modules in health care. Research using this kind of data has, for example, shown that healthcare trajectories are important for explaining the role the public views as appropriate for the government (Kikuzawa, Olafsdottir, & Pescosolido, 2008). Furthermore, it is possible to use these data to evaluate group differences in attitudes toward the healthcare system. An analysis of public attitudes in 33 countries showed that those in the labor force consistently evaluate the effectiveness of the healthcare system more negatively. However, the relationship between age and evaluations as well as education and evaluations is more mixed. For example, the more educated evaluate the healthcare system as more effective in 10 nations, as less effective in seven nations, with the remaining nations showing an insignificant relationship (Pescosolido & Olafsdottir, 2010). Healthcare systems have also been evaluated using Afrobarometer data, which include items on distance to health clinics, a major factor in healthcare inequities in rural Africa (Brinkerhoff, Wetterberg, & Wibbels, 2018).

While comparability is of course an issue regarding both types of data, the organizations (e.g., OECD, ISSP) responsible for these data implement specific strategies to increase comparability. This is done through cooperation between researchers across national contexts and careful translations of the instruments used in survey research. While many individual researchers interested in cross-national research rely on data that are centrally collected and distributed, comparability must not be taken for granted. Utilizing multiple measures, and paying attention to relative and absolute inequalities, are two strategies to assess robustness to assumptions about measurement comparability.

Finally, the relationship between theory and data is perhaps especially important in cross-national research, as theory can guide the research efforts and make sense of the observed patterns. This emphasis moves our efforts from showing that there are cross-national differences in healthcare disparities to allowing us to understand and explain why these cross-national differences may exist and how they relate to the institutional arrangements, historical trajectories, and cultural traditions of each country. The institutional framework developed in this book is one attempt to guide such inquiry.

Timing

While the strengths of comparative research include its ability to identify the institutional correlates of healthcare disparities and place healthcare disparities into a broader context, such research also faces the challenge of analyzing causal mechanisms in divergent settings. The inability to examine processes inside the "black boxes" theorized to connect cause and effect is related to the problem of complex lag structures, where an institutional change at time t may not affect the outcome until t + 1, 2, 3, etc. Fortunately, insights from social epidemiology about the etiology of different diseases and causes of death across the lifecourse can be useful in designing and testing rigorous hypotheses about the political-sociological factors that contribute to changing inequalities over time (Miech, Shanahan, Boardman, & Bauldry, 2015; Miech, Pampel, Kim, & Rogers, 2011).

A critical factor in the timing of effects of political-sociological exposures would be the unequal time horizons and uncertainty calculations made by people when considering health-relevant behaviors that depend on material resources, such as the timing of childbearing in developing countries (Trinitapoli & Yeatman, 2011). Embodiment happens over the lifecourse, raising questions about how political-sociological exposures might contribute to cumulative advantage processes that generate health inequities through "path- and duration-dependent processes" (Willson, Shuey, & Elder, 2007). As evidence on long-term trends in health inequities accumulates, a promising approach to estimating lagged, short-run, and long-run effects might draw on dynamic regression models for the analysis of time-series data (De Boef & Keele, 2008).

Independence

Many statistical techniques rely on the assumption that the cases analyzed are independent, but this is not a reasonable assumption where the cases are nation-states or other non-independent geographical areas such as the 50 states of the United States, neighborhoods in a metropolitan area, or cities in the same geographic region. This problem is perhaps more problematic than ever in the so-called era of globalization, which finds national societies deeply embedded in transnational networks. At the macro level, research can include information about network ties between polities by drawing on resources such as the Correlates of War data. At the individual level, promising and underutilized resources for the examination of how health depends on social relations that are potentially structured by political-sociological exposures include the Mexican Migration Project, Nang Rong Surveys, and (U.S.) National Longitudinal Study of Adolescent Health.

Space and Place

Climate change is the contemporary phenomenon with perhaps the largest long-term impact on the global distribution of population health. As the wavelike, amplified echo of industrialization, climate change shares some challenging properties with industrialization, including unintended consequences for socio-spatial organization, social stratification, and the materiality of places. This most macro-level of exposures will be channeled through politics and policy in its health effects, such as through citizenship laws, institutional boundaries, and the distribution of resources for adaptation. For instance, land and water rights are fundamental to the nation-state, and as the quantity and quality of these ecological elements change, political problems and novel political solutions will emerge. New work on adaptability to temperature change implies that demands for adaptation resources may cross existing political boundaries (Noelke et al., 2016). At the meso and micro levels of socio-political exposures, the neighborhoods and organizations where people live, learn, and work powerfully determine the distribution of health (Feldman et al., 2015; Massey & Denton, 1993; Pettit & Hook, 2009; Sampson, 2012).

Conclusion

While this chapter necessarily focuses on the challenges to interdisciplinary engagement between political sociology and social epidemiology, there is great promise in such engagement (Birn, 2009a; Ottersen et al., 2014). The core significance of such an effort, if successful, would be to develop a more epidemiological study of politics, and a more political study of epidemiology, by identifying and evaluating the political causes of the (very) uneven distribution of population health. Given the push from ecosocial, fundamental-cause, and social-determinants theories of disease distribution for concepts and measures for investigating politics and policies, the macroscope of political sociology holds great promise for generating new questions, new answers, and even new accountability for the generation of health inequity. At the same time, engagement with social-epidemiological concepts of etiologic period, population, and distribution offer political sociologists new and fruitful ways of thinking about how the rules of the game distribute valued social goods beyond income and wealth.

I close this short book with the hope that it spurs more collaboration between social epidemiologists and political sociologists as we engage urgent puzzles about the global distribution of population health. The first puzzle is the finding of a growing mortality gap between the United States and other rich democracies: a recent National Academy of Sciences report calls for new research on political factors that may contribute to this growing gap (Woolf & Aron, 2013). The second puzzle is the finding that Scandinavian welfare states, which have some of the more generous public welfare benefits in the world, also have some of the larger relative social inequities in health in the world: this "Nordic Paradox" is currently spurring large-scale research efforts and strong debate. The third puzzle is the relationship between the distribution of health within a population, and the average level of health of that population. Most generally, the finding of cross-national and historical variation in the patterning of health inequities represents arguably the foremost and broadest question that should engage scientists interested in the people's health.

BIBLIOGRAPHY

Alderson, A. S., & Nielsen, F. (2002). Globalization and the great U-turn: Income inequality trends in 16 OECD countries. *American Journal of Sociology, 107*(5), 1244–1299. https://doi.org/10.1086/341329

Alesina, A., Devleeschauwer, A., Easterly, W., Kurlat, S., & Wacziarg, R. (2003). Fractionalization. *Journal of Economic Growth, 8*(2), 155–194.

Amenta, E. (2000). *Bold Relief: Institutional Politics and the Origins of Modern American Social Policy.* Princeton, NJ: Princeton University Press.

Anand, S., Segal, P., & Stiglitz, J. (2010). *Debates on the measurement of global poverty.* Oxford, UK: Oxford University Press.

Anderson, B. (2006). *Imagined communities: Reflections on the origin and spread of nationalism.* London, UK: Verso Books.

Armstrong, D. A. (2011). Stability and change in the Freedom House political rights and civil liberties measures. *Journal of Peace Research, 48*(5), 653–662.

Atkinson, A. B. (1996). *Public Economics in Action: The Basic Income / Flat Tax Proposal.* Oxford, UK: Oxford University Press.

Atkinson, A. B., Rainwater, L., & Smeeding, T. M. (1995). Income distribution in advanced economies: Evidence from the Luxembourg Income Study (LIS). Luxembourg Income Study. Retrieved from http://www.lisdatacenter.org/wps/liswps/120.pdf

Avendano, M., Berkman, L. F., Brugiavini, A., & Pasini, G. (2015). The long-run effect of maternity leave benefits on mental health: Evidence from European countries. *Social Science and Medicine, 132*, 45–53. https://doi.org/10.1016/j.socscimed.2015.02.037

Bail, C. A. (2014). The cultural environment: Measuring culture with big data. *Theory and Society*, *43*(3–4), 465–482.

Bambra, C., Netuveli, G., & Eikemo, T. A. (2010). Welfare state regime life courses: the development of Western European welfare state regimes and age-related patterns of educational inequalities in self-reported health. *International Journal of Health Services*, *40*(3), 399–420.

Bartley, M. (2003). Commentary: Relating social structure and health. *International Journal of Epidemiology*, *32*(6), 958–960. https://doi.org/10.1093/ije/dyg232

Bauböck, R., & Guiraudon, V. (2009). Introduction: realignments of citizenship: reassessing rights in the age of plural memberships and multi-level governance. *Citizenship Studies*, *13*(5), 439–450. https://doi.org/10.1080/13621020903174613

Bearman, P. S., Moody, J., & Stovel, K. (2004). Chains of affection: The structure of adolescent romantic and sexual networks. *American Journal of Sociology*, *110*(1), 44–91.

Beckfield, J. (2003). Inequality in the world polity: The structure of international organization. *American Sociological Review*, *68*(3), 401–424.

Beckfield, J. (2004). Does income inequality harm health? New cross-national evidence. *Journal of Health and Social Behavior*, *45*(3), 231–248.

Beckfield, J. (2010). The social structure of the world polity. *American Journal of Sociology*, *115*(4), 1018–1068.

Beckfield, J. (2013). The end of equality in Europe? *Current History*, *112*(752), 94.

Beckfield, J., & Bambra, C. (2016). Shorter lives in stingier states: Social policy shortcomings help explain the US mortality disadvantage. *Social Science and Medicine*, *171*, 30–38. https://doi.org/10.1016/j.socscimed.2016.10.017

Beckfield, J., Bambra, C., Eikemo, T. A., Huijts, T., McNamara, C., & Wendt, C. (2015). An institutional theory of welfare state effects on the distribution of population health. *Social Theory and Health*, *13*(3–4), 227–244. https://doi.org/10.1057/sth.2015.19

Beckfield, J., & Krieger, N. (2009). Epi+ demos+ cracy: linking political systems and priorities to the magnitude of health inequities—evidence, gaps, and a research agenda. *Epidemiologic Reviews*, *31*(1), 152–177.

Beckfield, J., Olafsdottir, S., & Bakhtiari, E. (2013). Health inequalities in global context. *American Behavioral Scientist*, *57*(8), 1014–1039.

Beckfield, J., Olafsdottir, S., & Sosnaud, B. (2013). Healthcare systems in comparative perspective: Classification, convergence, institutions, inequalities, and five missed turns. *Annual Review of Sociology*, *39*, 127–146.

Beine, M., Boucher, A., Burgoon, B., Crock, M., Gest, J., Hiscox, M., Thielemann, E. (2016). Comparing immigration policies: An overview from the IMPALA database. *International Migration Review*, *50*(4), 827–863. https://doi.org/10.1111/imre.12169

Benefits and Wages: Tax-Benefit Calculator—OECD. (n.d.). Retrieved February 11, 2017, from http://www.oecd.org/els/soc/benefitsandwagestax-benefitcalculator.htm.

Berezin, M. (2002). Secure states: towards a political sociology of emotion. *The Sociological Review*, *50*(S2), 33–52.

Berezin, M. (2009). Illiberal politics in neoliberal times. *Culture, Security and Populism in the New Europe.* Cambridge, UK: Cambridge University Press. Retrieved from http://www.langtoninfo.com/web_content/9780521547840_frontmatter.pdf

Berkman, L. F., Kawachi, I., & Glymour, M. (2014). *Social Epidemiology*. New York, NY: Oxford University Press.

Bird, C. E., & Rieker, P. P. (2008). *Gender and Health: The Effects of Constrained Choices and Social Policies*. New York, NY: Cambridge University Press.

Birn, A.-E. (2009a). Making it politic(al): closing the gap in a generation: health equity through action on the social determinants of health. *Social Medicine*, *4*(3), 166–182.

Birn, A.-E. (2009b). *Textbook of international health: global health in a dynamic world*. New York, NY: Oxford University Press.

Blakely, T., Lynch, J., & Bentley, R. (2016). Commentary: DAGs and the restricted potential outcomes approach are tools, not theories of causation. *International Journal of Epidemiology*, *45*(6), 1835–1837.

Bonikowski, B. (2010). Cross-national interaction and cultural similarity: A relational analysis. *International Journal of Comparative Sociology*, *51*(5), 315–348. https://doi.org/10.1177/0020715210376854

Brady, D. & Amie Bostic. (2015). Paradoxes of social policy: welfare transfers, relative poverty, and redistribution preferences. *American Sociological Review*, *80*(2), 268–298. https://doi.org/10.1177/0003122415573049

Brady, D., Blome, A., & Kleider, H. (2016). How politics and institutions shape poverty and inequality. *The Oxford Handbook of the Social Science of Poverty*, New York, NY: Oxford University Press.

Brady, D., & Finnigan, R. (2014). Does immigration undermine public support for social policy? *American Sociological Review*, *79*(1), 17–42.

Brady, D., Finnigan, R. M., & Hübgen, S. (2017). Rethinking the risks of poverty: a framework for analyzing prevalences and penalties. *American Journal of Sociology*, *123*(3), 740–786.

Brady, D., Huber, E., & Stephens, J. D. (2016). Comparative welfare states data set, 2014. LIS Data Center. Retrieved from http://www.lisdatacenter.org/wp-content/uploads/CWS-codebook.pdf.

Brand, J. E., & Xie, Y. (2010). Who benefits most from college? Evidence for negative selection in heterogeneous economic returns to higher education. *American Sociological Review*, *75*(2), 273–302. https://doi.org/10.1177/0003122410363567

Breen, R., Choi, S., & Holm, A. (2015). Heterogeneous causal effects and sample selection bias. *Sociological Science*, *2*, 351–369.

Brinkerhoff, D. W., Wetterberg, A., & Wibbels, E. (2018). Distance, services, and citizen perceptions of the state in rural Africa. *Governance*, *31*(1), 103–124. https://doi.org/10.1111/gove.12271

Brooks, C., & Manza, J. (2008). *Why welfare states persist: The importance of public opinion in democracies*. Chicago, IL: University of Chicago Press. Retrieved from https://books.google.com.ni/books?hl=en&lr=&id=zRVNMu74dB8C&oi=fnd&pg=PR5&dq=comparative+welfare+states+dataset&ots=MzmczRe0vk&sig=2SiE6vJ69V7sbUZKvh_oHWhCr4s.

Bryant, T., & Raphael, D. (2005). Politics, public policy, and population health in the United Kingdom. *UK Health Watch 2005: The Experience of Health in an Unequal Society*, 15–22. ISBN 1 874038 76 7.

Burstein, P. (1991). Policy domains: Organization, culture, and policy outcomes. *Annual Review of Sociology*, *17*(1), 327–350.

Campbell, A. L. (2014). *Trapped in America's Safety Net: One Family's Struggle*. Chicago, IL: University of Chicago Press. Retrieved from https://books. google.com.ni/books?hl=en&lr=&id=UOYvBAAAQBAJ&oi=fnd& pg=PR7&dq=andrea+campbell+america%27s+safety+net&ots=od-3u7u6fn&sig=8QGRxQHeVFJNJe121_psxQF6d8s.

Chen, F., Yang, Y., & Liu, G. (2010). Social change and socioeconomic disparities in health over the life course in China: a cohort analysis. *American Sociological Review*, *75*(1), 126–150. https://doi.org/10.1177/0003122409359165

Chorev, N. (2012). *The World Health Organization between North and South*. Ithaca, NY: Cornell University Press.

Clark, R. (2010). Technical and institutional states: Loose coupling in the human rights sector of the world polity. *The Sociological Quarterly*, *51*(1), 65–95.

Clemens, E. S. (2007). Toward a historicized sociology: Theorizing events, processes, and emergence. *Annual Review of Sociology*, *33*, 527–549.

Clemens, E. S. (2016). *What Is Political Sociology?* Cambridge, UK: Polity Press.

Clemens, E. S., & Cook, J. M. (1999). Politics and institutionalism: Explaining durability and change. *Annual Review of Sociology*, *25*, 441–466.

Conley, D., & Springer, K. W. (2001). Welfare state and infant mortality. *American Journal of Sociology*, *107*(3), 768–807. https://doi.org/10.1086/338781

Coppedge, M., Gerring, J., Lindberg, S., Skaaning, S.-E., Teorell, J., Andersson, F., Wang, Y. (2016). V-Dem Methodology V6 (SSRN Scholarly Paper No. ID 2951040). Rochester, NY: Social Science Research Network. Retrieved from https://papers.ssrn.com/abstract=2951040.

Crane, J. T. (2013). *Scrambling for Africa: AIDS, expertise, and the rise of American global health science*. Ithaca, NY: Cornell University Press. Retrieved from https://books.google.com/books?hl=en&lr=&id=zY2vA AAAQBAJ&oi=fnd&pg=PR7&dq=scrambling+for+africa&ots=KZn6 cnVfbs&sig=r2vpWQpMdJjbSc4akSEGld4Dxag.

Curran, S. R., Garip, F., Chung, C. Y., & Tangchonlatip, K. (2005). Gendered migrant social capital: Evidence from Thailand. *Social Forces*, *84*(1), 225.

Cutler, D. (2004). *Your Money or Your Life: Strong Medicine for America's Health Care System*. New York, NY: Oxford University Press.

Cutler, D. M., Deaton, A. S., & Lleras-Muney, A. (2006). *The determinants of mortality*. Cambridge, MA: National Bureau of Economic Research.

Davey Smith, G. (2011). Epidemiology, epigenetics and the 'Gloomy Prospect': embracing randomness in population health research and practice. *International Journal of Epidemiology*, 40(3), 537–562.

Davey Smith, G., Gorter, A., Hoppenbrouwer, J., Sweep, A., Perez, R. M., Gonzales, C., Morales, P., Pauw, J., & Sandiford, P. (1993). The cultural construction of childhood diarrhea in rural Nicaragua: relevance for epidemiology and health promotion. *Social Science & Medicine*, 36(12), 1613–1624.

Davey Smith, G., Relton, C. L., & Brennan, P. (2016). Chance, choice and cause in cancer aetiology: individual and population perspectives. *International Journal of Epidemiology*, 45(1), 605–613.

Davidov, E., Meuleman, B., Cieciuch, J., Schmidt, P., & Billiet, J. (2014). Measurement equivalence in cross-national research. *Annual Review of Sociology*, 40, 55–75.

Davis, G. F., McAdam, D., Scott, W. R., & Zald, M. N. (2005). *Social Movements and Organization Theory*. New York, NY: Cambridge University Press.

De Boef, S., & Keele, L. (2008). Taking time seriously. *American Journal of Political Science*, 52(1), 184–200.

DiMaggio, P., & Garip, F. (2012). Network effects and social inequality. *Annual Review of Sociology*, 38, 93–118.

Dobbin, F. (1994). *Forging Industrial Policy: The United States, Britain, and France in the Railway Age*. New York, NY: Cambridge University Press.

Durkheim, É. (1938 [1895]). *The Rules of Sociological Method*. New York, NY: Free Press.

Earl, J., & Kimport, K. (2011). *Digitally enabled social change: Activism in the internet age*. Cambridge, MA: MIT Press.

Ebbinghaus, B. (2005). When less is more: Selection problems in large-N and small-N cross-national comparisons. *International Sociology*, 20(2), 133–152.

Eikemo, T. A., Balaj, M., Bambra, C., Beckfield, J., Huijts, T., and McNamara, C. L., Eds. (2017). *Social Inequalities in Health and Their Deteriminants*. Supplement to the *European Journal of Public Health*, 27(Suppl. 1).

Eikemo, T. A., & Bambra, C. (2008). The welfare state: a glossary for public health. *Journal of Epidemiology and Community Health*, *62*(1), 3–6. https://doi.org/10.1136/jech.2007.066787

Esping-Andersen, G. (1990). *The Three Worlds of Welfare Capitalism*. Princeton, NJ: Princeton University Press.

Esping-Andersen, G., & Korpi, W. (1986). From poor relief to institutional welfare states: the development of Scandinavian social policy. *International Journal of Sociology*, *16*(3/4), 39–74.

Esping-Andersen, G. (2002). A child-centred social investment strategy. In G. Esping-Andersen, D. Gallie, A. Hemerijck, & J. Myles, (Eds.), *Why We Need a New Welfare State* (pp. 26–67). Oxford, UK: Oxford University Press.

Evans, W. N., Hout, M., & Mayer, S. E. (2004). Assessing the effect of economic inequality. In K. Neckerman (Ed.), *Social Inequality* (pp. 933–968). New York, NY: Russell Sage Foundation.

Fearon, J. D. (2003). Ethnic and cultural diversity by country. *Journal of Economic Growth*, *8*(2), 195–222.

Feldman, J. M., Waterman, P. D., Coull, B. A., & Krieger, N. (2015). Spatial social polarisation: using the Index of Concentration at the Extremes jointly for income and race/ethnicity to analyse risk of hypertension. *Journal of Epidemiology and Community Health*, *69*(12), 1199–1207.

Ferraro, K. F., & Shippee, T. P. (2009). Aging and cumulative inequality: How does inequality get under the skin? *The Gerontologist*, *49*(3), 333–343.

Ferrera, M. (2005). *The Boundaries of Welfare: European Integration and the New Spatial Politics of Social Protection*. Oxford, UK: Oxford University Press.

Fligstein, N. (2001). Social skill and the theory of fields. *Sociological Theory*, *19*(2), 105–125.

Fligstein, N., & McAdam, D. (2012). *A theory of fields*. New York, NY: Oxford University Press.

Forget, E. L. (2011). The town with no poverty: The health effects of a Canadian guaranteed annual income field experiment. *Canadian Public Policy*, *37*(3), 283–305.

Freese, J., & Kevern, J. A. (2013). Types of causes. In S. L. Morgan (Ed.), *Handbook of Causal Analysis for Social Research* (pp. 27–41). Netherlands: Springer. https://doi.org/10.1007/978-94-007-6094-3_3

Gage-Bouchard, E. A. (2017). Culture, styles of institutional interactions, and inequalities in healthcare experiences. *Journal of Health and Social Behavior*, *58*(2), 147–165. https://doi.org/10.1177/0022146517693051

Garip, F. (2008). Social capital and migration: How do similar resources lead to divergent outcomes? *Demography*, *45*(3), 591–617.

Garriga, A. C. (2016). Central bank independence in the world: a new data set. *International Interactions*, *42*(5), 849–868. https://doi.org/10.1080/03050629.2016.1188813

Gauri, V., & Lieberman, E. S. (2006). Boundary institutions and HIV/AIDS policy in Brazil and South Africa. *Studies in Comparative International Development*, *41*(3), 47.

Gerstle, G., & Mollenkopf, J. (2001). *E pluribus unum?: contemporary and historical perspectives on immigrant political incorporation*. New York, NY: Russell Sage Foundation.

Gkiouleka, A., Huijts, T., Beckfield, J., & Bambra, C. (2018). Understanding the micro and macro politics of health: Inequalities, intersectionality & institutions-A research agenda. *Social Science & Medicine*, *200*, 92–98.

Glenn, E. N. (2011). Constructing citizenship exclusion, subordination, and resistance. *American Sociological Review*, *76*(1), 1–24. https://doi.org/10.1177/0003122411398443

Go, J. (2013). For a postcolonial sociology. *Theory and Society*, *42*(1), 25–55. https://doi.org/10.1007/s11186-012-9184-6

Goesling, B., & Firebaugh, G. (2004). The trend in international health inequality. *Population and Development Review*, *30*(1), 131–146. https://doi.org/10.1111/j.1728-4457.2004.00006.x

Goldberg, A. D., Allis, C. D., & Bernstein, E. (2007). Epigenetics: A landscape takes shape. *Cell*, *128*(4), 635–638. https://doi.org/10.1016/j.cell.2007.02.006

Gross, N. (2009). A pragmatist theory of social mechanisms. *American Sociological Review*, *74*(3), 358–379.

Grusky, D. B. (2001). Social stratification: Class, race, and gender in sociological perspective. Retrieved from http://ecsocman.hse.ru/text/19153213/.

Hacker, D. (2017). *Legalized Families in the Era of Bordered Globalization.* New York, NY: Cambridge University Press.

Hacker, J. S. (2002). *The Divided Welfare State: The Battle Over Public and Private Social Benefits in the United States.* New York, NY: Cambridge University Press.

Hafner-Burton, E. M., & Tsutsui, K. (2005). Human rights in a globalizing world: The paradox of empty promises. *American Journal of Sociology, 110*(5), 1373–1411.

Halaby, C. N. (2004). Panel models in sociological research: Theory into practice. *Annual Review of Sociology, 30*(1), 507–544.

Hall, P. A., & Lamont, M. (2009). *Successful societies: How institutions and culture affect health.* New York, NY: Cambridge University Press.

Hall, P. A., & Soskice, D. (2001). *Varieties of Capitalism: The Institutional Foundations of Comparative Advantage.* New York, NY: Oxford University Press.

Hall, P. A., & Taylor, R. C. R. (1996). Political science and the three new institutionalisms. *Political Studies, 44*(5), 936–957.

Han, C., & Whyte, M. K. (2009). The social contours of distributive injustice feelings in contemporary China. In Davis, D., & Wang, F., Eds. *Creating Wealth and Poverty in Postsocialist China* (pp. 193–212). Stanford, CA: Stanford University Press.

Han, D. (2010). Policing and racialization of rural migrant workers in Chinese cities. *Ethnic and Racial Studies, 33*(4), 593–610. https://doi.org/10.1080/01419870903325651

Harris, J. (2017). *Achieving Access: Professional Movements and the Politics of Health Universalism.* Ithaca, NY: Cornell University Press.

Hatzenbuehler, M. L. (2009). How does sexual minority stigma "get under the skin"? A psychological mediation framework. *Psychological Bulletin, 135*(5), 707.

Häusermann, S. (2006). Changing coalitions in social policy reforms: the politics of new social needs and demands. *Journal of European Social Policy, 16*(1), 5–21.

Häusermann, S., & Kriesi, H. (2011). What do voters want? Dimensions and configurations in individual-level preferences and party choice. In *Conference on the Future of Democratic Capitalism*, June 16–18, 2011, Zurich.

Hedström, P., & Bearman, P. (2009). *The Oxford handbook of analytical sociology*. New York, NY: Oxford University Press.

Heijmans, B. T., & Mill, J. (2012). Commentary: The seven plagues of epigenetic epidemiology. *International Journal of Epidemiology*, *41*(1), 74–78. https://doi.org/10.1093/ije/dyr225

Hertzman, C., & Boyce, T. (2010). How experience gets under the skin to create gradients in developmental health. *Annual Review of Public Health*, *31*, 329–347.

Hochschild, J. L., & Mollenkopf, J. H. (2009). *Bringing outsiders in: Transatlantic perspectives on immigrant political incorporation*. Ithaca, NY: Cornell University Press.

Huber, E., Ragin, C., & Stephens, J. D. (1993). Social democracy, Christian democracy, constitutional structure, and the welfare state. *American Journal of Sociology*, *99*(3), 711–749.

Huber, E., Ragin, C., & Stephens, J. D. (1997). Comparative welfare states data set.

Hung, H., & Thompson, D. (2016). Money supply, class power, and inflation: monetarism reassessed. *American Sociological Review*, *81*(3), 447–466. https://doi.org/10.1177/0003122416639609

Idler, E. L., & Benyamini, Y. (1997). Self-rated health and mortality: a review of twenty-seven community studies. *Journal of Health and Social Behavior*, *38*(1), 21–37. https://doi.org/10.2307/2955359

Immergut, E. M. (1990). Institutions, veto points, and policy results: A comparative analysis of health care. *Journal of Public Policy*, *10*(04), 391–416.

IMPALA Database —. (n.d.). Retrieved February 24, 2017, from http://www.impaladatabase.org/.

Internet TAXSIM Version 9. (n.d.). Retrieved February 11, 2017, from http://users.nber.org/~taxsim/taxsim9/.

Janoski, T., Alford, R. R., Hicks, A. M., & Schwartz, M. A. (Eds.). (2005). *The Handbook of Political Sociology: States, Civil Societies, and Globalization*. New York: Cambridge University Press.

Jen, M. H., Jones, K., & Johnston, R. (2009). Global variations in health: evaluating Wilkinson's income inequality hypothesis using the World Values Survey. *Social Science & Medicine, 68*(4), 643–653.

Jencks, C. (1972). Inequality: A reassessment of the effect of family and schooling in America. Retrieved from http://psycnet.apa.org/psycinfo/2003-00040-000.

Jenson, J. (1997). Fated to live in interesting times: canada's changing citizenship regimes. *Canadian Journal of Political Science, 30*(4), 627–644.

Kelly, M. P. (1980). *White-collar Proletariat: Industrial Behaviour of British Civil Servants*, London: Rutledge & Kegan Hall.

Kenworthy, L. (2004). *Egalitarian Capitalism: Jobs, Incomes, and Growth in Affluent Countries*. New York, NY: Russell Sage Foundation.

Kikuzawa, S., Olafsdottir, S., & Pescosolido, B. A. (2008). Similar pressures, different contexts: public attitudes toward government intervention for health care in 21 nations. *Journal of Health and Social Behavior, 49*(4), 385–399. https://doi.org/10.1177/002214650804900402

Killewald, A., & Gough, M. (2013). Does specialization explain marriage penalties and premiums? *American Sociological Review, 78*(3), 477–502.

Kim, D., Kawachi, I., Vander Hoorn, S., & Ezzati, M. (2008). Is inequality at the heart of it? Cross-country associations of income inequality with cardiovascular diseases and risk factors. *Social Science & Medicine, 66*(8), 1719–1732.

Korpi, W. (1983). *The democratic class struggle*. London, UK: Routledge.

Korpi, W., Ferrarini, T., & Englund, S. (2013). Women's opportunities under different family policy constellations: gender, class, and inequality tradeoffs in Western countries re-examined. *Social Politics: International Studies in Gender, State and Society, 20*(1), 1–40. https://doi.org/10.1093/sp/jxs028

Korpi, W., & Palme, J. (1998). The paradox of redistribution and strategies of equality: welfare state institutions, inequality, and poverty in the Western countries. *American Sociological Review*, *63*(5), 661–687. https://doi.org/ 10.2307/2657333

Krause, M. (2014). *The Good Project: Humanitarian Relief NGOs and the Fragmentation of Reason*. Chicago, IL: University of Chicago Press.

Krieger, N. (1994). Epidemiology and the web of causation: Has anyone seen the spider? *Social Science and Medicine*, *39*(7), 887–903. https://doi.org/ 10.1016/0277-9536(94)90202-X

Krieger, N. (2011). *Epidemiology and the people's health: theory and context,* Vol. 213. New York: Oxford University Press.

Krieger, N. (2012). Who and what is a "population"? Historical debates, current controversies, and implications for understanding "population health" and rectifying health inequities. *Milbank Quarterly*, *90*(4), 634–681. https:// doi.org/10.1111/j.1468-0009.2012.00678.x

Krieger, N., Chen, J. T., Coull, B. A., Beckfield, J., Kiang, M. V., & Waterman, P. D. (2014). Jim Crow and premature mortality among the US black and white population, 1960–2009: an age–period–cohort analysis. *Epidemiology*, *25*(4), 494.

Krieger, N., Chen, J. T., Coull, B., Waterman, P. D., & Beckfield, J. (2013). The unique impact of abolition of Jim Crow laws on reducing inequities in infant death rates and implications for choice of comparison groups in analyzing societal determinants of health. *American Journal of Public Health*, *103*(12), 2234–2244. https://doi.org/10.2105/AJPH.2013.301350

Krieger, N., & Davey Smith, G. (2016). The tale wagged by the DAG: broadening the scope of causal inference and explanation for epidemiology. *International Journal of Epidemiology*, *45*(6), 1787–1808.

Krieger, N., Rehkopf, D. H., Chen, J. T., Waterman, P. D., Marcelli, E., & Kennedy, M. (2008). The fall and rise of US inequities in premature mortality: 1960–2002. *PLoS Medicine*, *5*(2), e46.

Krieger, N., Singh, N., Chen, J. T., Coull, B. A., Beckfield, J., Kiang, M. V., & Gruskin, S. (2015). Why history matters for quantitative target setting: Long-term trends in socioeconomic and racial/ethnic inequities in U.S. infant death rates (1960–2010). *Journal of Public Health Policy*, *36*(3), 287–303.

Krieger, N., Waterman, P. D., Gryparis, A., & Coull, B. A. (2015). Black carbon exposure, socioeconomic and racial/ethnic spatial polarization, and the Index of Concentration at the Extremes (ICE). *Health and Place, 34,* 215–228.

Krippner, G. R. (2011). *Capitalizing on Crisis.* Cambridge, MA: Harvard University Press.

Kunitz, S. J. (2015). *Regional Cultures and Mortality in America.* New York, NY: Cambridge University Press.

Lareau, A. (2011). *Unequal childhoods: Class, race, and family life.* Berkeley and Los Angeles, CA: University of California Press.

Lee, J., & Bean, F. D. (2004). America's changing color lines: Immigration, race/ethnicity, and multiracial identification. *Annual Review of Sociology, 30,* 221–242.

Lee, J., & Bean, F. D. (2010). *The diversity paradox: Immigration and the color line in twenty-first century America.* New York, NY: Russell Sage Foundation.

Leicht, K. T., & Jenkins, J. C. (2011). *Handbook of Politics.* Springer. Retrieved from http://link.springer.com/content/pdf/10.1007/978-0-387-68930-2.pdf.

Lewis, K. (2013). The limits of racial prejudice. *Proceedings of the National Academy of Sciences, 110*(47), 18814–18819.

Lewis, K. (2015). Three fallacies of digital footprints. *Big Data and Society, 2*(2), 1–4.

Lieberman, E. S. (2005). Nested analysis as a mixed-method strategy for comparative research. *American Political Science Review, 99*(03), 435–452.

Lieberson, S. (1985). *Making it count: The improvement of social research and theory.* Berkeley and Los Angeles, CA: University of California Press.

Lieberson, S. (1991). Small N's and big conclusions: an examination of the reasoning in comparative studies based on a small number of cases. *Social Forces, 70*(2), 307–320.

Lijphart, A. (1995). *Electoral Systems and Party Systems.* New York: Oxford University Press, USA. Retrieved from http://library.nsa.gov.ng/handle/123456789/159.

Link, B. G., & Phelan, J. (1995). Social conditions as fundamental causes of disease. *Journal of Health and Social Behavior*, Supplement, 80–94.

Liu, K.-Y., King, M., & Bearman, P. S. (2010). Social influence and the autism epidemic. *American Journal of Sociology*, *115*(5), 1387–1434.

Lundberg, O., Yngwe, M. A., Bergqvist, K., & Sjoeberg, O. (2015). Welfare states and health inequalities. *Canadian Public Policy*, *41*(suppl. 2), S26–S33.

Lynch, J. (2008). The politics of territorial health inequalities in Europe. Presentation at the Annual Meeting of the American Political Science Association, August 28–31, 2008, Boston, MA.

Mackenbach, J. P., Kunst, A. E., Cavelaars, A. E., Groenhof, F., & Geurts, J. J. (1997). Socioeconomic inequalities in morbidity and mortality in Western Europe. *The Lancet*, *349*(9066), 1655–1659. https://doi.org/10.1016/S0140-6736(96)07226-1

Mahler, V. A., & Jesuit, D. K. (2006). Fiscal redistribution in the developed countries: new insights from the Luxembourg Income Study. *Socio-Economic Review*, *4*(3), 483–511. https://doi.org/10.1093/ser/mwl003

Mansbridge, J. (2003). Rethinking representation. *American Political Science Review*, *97*(4), 515–528. https://doi.org/10.1017/S0003055403000856

Marmot, M. (2005). Social determinants of health inequalities. *The Lancet*, *365*(9464), 1099–1104. https://doi.org/10.1016/S0140-6736(05)71146-6

Marmot, M., & Wilkinson, R. (2005). *Social Determinants of Health*. Oxford, UK: Oxford University Press.

Marshall, T. H. (1963). Citizenship and social class. *Sociology at the Crossroads*, 67–127. London, UK: Heinemann.

Massey, D. S. (2009). Racial formation in theory and practice: The case of Mexicans in the United States. *Race and Social Problems*, *1*(1), 12–26.

Massey, D. S., & Denton, N. A. (1993). *American apartheid: Segregation and the making of the underclass*. Cambridge, MA: Harvard University Press.

McAdam, D. (1990). *Freedom Summer*. New York, NY: Oxford University Press.

McCabe, J., Fairchild, E., Grauerholz, L., Pescosolido, B. A., & Tope, D. (2011). Gender in twentieth-century children's books: Patterns of disparity in titles and central characters. *Gender and Society*, *25*(2), 197–226.

McDade, T. W., Williams, S., & Snodgrass, J. J. (2007). What a drop can do: dried blood spots as a minimally invasive method for integrating biomarkers into population-based research. *Demography*, *44*(4), 899–925.

McDonnell, E. M. (2015). "Weberian bureaucracy and health: Does bureaucratic state capacity improve wellbeing?" Presentation at the annual meeting of the American Sociological Association.

McDonnell, E. M. (2016). Conciliatory states: Elite ethno-demographics and the puzzle of public goods within diverse African states. *Comparative Political Studies*, *49*(11), 1513–1549.

McDonnell, T. E. (2014). Drawing out culture: productive methods to measure cognition and resonance. *Theory and Society*, *43*(3–4), 247–274.

McEwen, B. S. (2012). Brain on stress: how the social environment gets under the skin. *Proceedings of the National Academy of Sciences*, *109*(Suppl 2), 17180–17185.

McKeown, T. (2014 [1979]). *The Role of Medicine: Dream, Mirage, or Nemesis?* Princeton, NJ: Princeton University Press.

McKinlay, J. B., & McKinlay, S. M. (1977). The questionable contribution of medical measures to the decline of mortality in the United States in the twentieth century. *The Milbank Memorial Fund Quarterly. Health and Society*, *55*(3), 405–428. https://doi.org/10.2307/3349539

Meyer, J. W. (2010). World society, institutional theories, and the actor. *Annual Review of Sociology*, *36*, 1–20.

Meyer, J. W., Boli, J., Thomas, G. M., & Ramirez, F. O. (1997). World society and the nation-state. *American Journal of Sociology*, *103*(1), 144–181.

Meyer, J. W., Tyack, D., Nagel, J., & Gordon, A. (1979). Public education as nation-building in America: enrollments and bureaucratization in the American states, 1870–1930. *American Journal of Sociology*, *85*(3), 591–613.

Midgley, J. (1999). Growth, redistribution, and welfare: Toward social investment. *Social Service Review*, *73*(1), 3–21.

Miech, R. A., Shanahan, M. J., Boardman, J., & Bauldry, S. (2015). The sequencing of a college degree during the transition to adulthood: Implications for obesity. *Journal of Health and Social Behavior*, *56*(2), 281–295.

Miech, R., Pampel, F., Kim, J., & Rogers, R. G. (2011). The enduring association between education and mortality: the role of widening and narrowing disparities. *American Sociological Review*, *76*(6), 913–934.

Migrant Integration Policy Index | MIPEX 2015. (2015) Retrieved February 24, 2017, from http://www.mipex.eu/.

Miller, G. (2008). Women's suffrage, political responsiveness, and child survival in American history. *The Quarterly Journal of Economics*, *123*(3), 1287–1327. https://doi.org/10.1162/qjec.2008.123.3.1287

Misra, J., Budig, M., & Boeckmann, I. (2011). Work-family policies and the effects of children on women's employment hours and wages. *Community, Work and Family*, *14*(2), 139–157. https://doi.org/10.1080/13668803.2011.571396

Mohr, J. W., & Ghaziani, A. (2014). Problems and prospects of measurement in the study of culture. *Theory and Society*, *43*(3–4), 225–246. https://doi.org/10.1007/s11186-014-9227-2

Moller, S., Alderson, A. S., & Nielsen, F. (2009). Changing patterns of income inequality in U.S. counties, 1970–2000. *American Journal of Sociology*, *114*(4), 1037–1101. https://doi.org/10.1086/595943

Monk Jr., E. P. (2016). The consequences of "race and color" in Brazil. *Social Problems*, *63*(3), 413–430.

Morel, N., Palier, B., & Palme, J. (2012). *Towards a social investment welfare state? ideas, policies and challenges*. Bristol, UK: Policy Press.

Morgan, K. J. (2006). *Working Mothers and the Welfare State: Religion and the Politics of Work-Family Policies in Western Europe and the United States*. Stanford, CA: Stanford University Press.

Morgan, K. J., & Zippel, K. (2003). Paid to care: the origins and effects of care leave policies in Western Europe. *Social Politics: International Studies in Gender, State and Society*, *10*(1), 49–85. https://doi.org/10.1093/sp/jxg004

Morris, A. (1981). Black Southern student sit-in movement: an analysis of internal organization. *American Sociological Review*, *46*(6), 744–767. https://doi.org/10.2307/2095077

Newey, C., Nolte, E., McKee, M., & Mossialos, E. (2003). Avoidable mortality in the enlarged European Union. Institute Des Sciences et de Sante, Paris. Retrieved from https://www.researchgate.net/profile/Elias_Mossialos/publication/228988065_Avoidable_mortality_in_the_enlarged_European_Union/links/5557e59708ae6943a874c282.pdf.

Noelke, C., & Beckfield, J. (2014). Recessions, job loss, and mortality among older U.S. adults. *American Journal of Public Health*, *104*(11), e126–e134. https://doi.org/10.2105/AJPH.2014.302210

Noelke, C., McGovern, M., Corsi, D. J., Jimenez, M. P., Stern, A., Wing, I. S., & Berkman, L. (2016). Increasing ambient temperature reduces emotional well-being. *Environmental Research*, *151*, 124–129.

Oakes, J. M., & Kaufman, J. S. (2006). *Methods in Social Epidemiology*. New York: John Wiley & Sons.

Olafsdottir, S. (2007). Fundamental causes of health disparities: stratification, the welfare state, and health in the United States and Iceland. *Journal of Health and Social Behavior*, *48*(3), 239–253.

Omi, M., & Winant, H. (2014). *Racial Formation in the United States*. London, UK: Routledge.

Orloff, A. S. (1993). Gender and the social rights of citizenship: the comparative analysis of gender relations and welfare states. *American Sociological Review*, *58*(3), 303–328. https://doi.org/10.2307/2095903

Osypuk, T. L., Joshi, P., Geronimo, K., & Acevedo-Garcia, D. (2014). Do social and economic policies influence health? A review. *Current Epidemiology Reports*, *1*(3), 149–164. https://doi.org/10.1007/s40471-014-0013-5

Ottersen, O. P., Dasgupta, J., Blouin, C., Buss, P., Chongsuvivatwong, V., . . . Frenk, J. (2014). The political origins of health inequity: prospects for change. *The Lancet*, *383*(9917), 630–667.

Pager, D. (2003). The mark of a criminal record. *American Journal of Sociology*, *108*(5), 937–975.

Pager, D., & Quillian, L. (2005). Walking the talk? What employers say versus what they do. *American Sociological Review, 70*(3), 355–380.

Pager, D., Western, B., & Bonikowski, B. (2009). Discrimination in a low-wage labor market: A field experiment. *American Sociological Review, 74*(5), 777–799.

Pescosolido, B. A., & Olafsdottir, S. (2010). The cultural turn in sociology: Can it help us resolve an age-old problem in understanding decision making for health care? *Sociological Forum, 25*(4), 655–676.

Pettit, B., & Hook, J. L. (2009). *Gendered Tradeoffs: Women, Family, and Workplace Inequality in Twenty-One Countries.* New York, NY: Russell Sage Foundation.

Pevehouse, J., Nordstrom, T., & Warnke, K. (2004). The Correlates of War 2: international Governmental Organizations Data version 2.0. *Conflict Management and Peace Science, 21*(2), 101–119.

Pierson, P. (1993). When effect becomes cause: Policy feedback and political change. *World Politics, 45*(04), 595–628.

Pierson, P. (2004). *Politics in time: History, institutions, and social analysis.* Princeton, NJ: Princeton University Press.

Pinto, S., & Beckfield, J. (2011). Organized labor in European countries, 1960–2006: persistent diversity and shared decline. *Research in the Sociology of Work, 22,* 153–179.

Pontusson, J. (2005). *Inequality and Prosperity: Social Europe vs. Liberal America.* Ithaca, NY: Cornell University Press.

Posner, D. N. (2004). Measuring ethnic fractionalization in Africa. *American Journal of Political Science, 48*(4), 849–863.

Powell, W. W., & DiMaggio, P. J. (2012). *The New Institutionalism in Organizational Analysis.* Chicago, IL: University of Chicago Press.

Prasad, M. (2012). *The Land of Too Much: American Abundance and the Paradox of Poverty.* Cambridge, MA: Harvard University Press.

Quality of Government (QOG), University of Gothenburg, Sweden. (n.d.). Retrieved November 24, 2016, from http://qog.pol.gu.se/

Quesnel-Vallée, A. (2007). Self-rated health: caught in the crossfire of the quest for "true" health? *International Journal of Epidemiology, 36*(6), 1161–1164. https://doi.org/10.1093/ije/dym236

Ramage, D., Dumais, S. T., & Liebling, D. J. (2010). Characterizing microblogs with topic models. Presentation at the International Conference on Weblogs and Social Media, May 23–26, 2010, Washington, DC.

Ratcliff, K. S. (2017). *The Social Determinants of Health: Looking Upstream.* Cambridge, UK; Malden, MA: Polity.

Ray, R., Brown, M., Fraistat, N., & Summers, E. (2017). Ferguson and the death of Michael Brown on Twitter: #BlackLivesMatter, #TCOT, and the evolution of collective identities. *Ethnic and Racial Studies, 40*(11), 1797–1813.

Reardon, S. F., & Bischoff, K. (2011). *American Journal of Sociology, 116*(4), 1092–1153. https://doi.org/10.1086/657114

Reibling, N., & Wendt, C. (2012). Gatekeeping and provider choice in OECD healthcare systems. *Current Sociology, 60*(4), 489–505.

Reibling, N., & Wendt, C. (2013). Regulating patients' access to healthcare services. In Mervio, M., Ed. *Healthcare Management and Economics: Perspectives on Public and Private Administration* (pp. 53–68). Hershey, PA: Medical Information Science Reference.

Relton, C. L., & Smith, G. D. (2010). Epigenetic epidemiology of common complex disease: prospects for prediction, prevention, and treatment. *PLOS Medicine, 7*(10), e1000356. https://doi.org/10.1371/journal.pmed.1000356

Reynolds, M. M., & Brady, D. (2012). Bringing you more than the weekend: union membership and self-rated health in the United States. *Social Forces, 90*(3), 1023–1049.

Riley, J. C. (2001). *Rising Life Expectancy: A Global History.* New York, NY: Cambridge University Press.

Robins, J. M., & Weissman, M. B. (2016). Commentary: Counterfactual causation and streetlamps: what is to be done? *International Journal of Epidemiology, 45*(6), 1830–1835.

Robinson, R. S. (2015). Population policy in sub-Saharan Africa: A case of both normative and coercive ties to the world polity. *Population Research and Policy Review, 34*(2), 201–221. https://doi.org/10.1007/s11113-014-9338-5

Rodriguez, J. M., Bound, J., & Geronimus, A. T. (2014). U.S. infant mortality and the president's party. *International Journal of Epidemiology, 43*(3), 818–826.

Rodríguez-Muñiz, M. (2016) *Figures of the Future: National Latino Civil Rights Advocacy and the Politics of Demography*. PhD Dissertation, Brown University, Providence, RI.

Rothman, K. J., Greenland, S., & Lash, T. L. (2008). *Modern Epidemiology*. New York, NY: Lippincott Williams & Wilkins.

Rothstein, B. (2011). *The quality of government: Corruption, social trust, and inequality in international perspective*. Chicago, IL: University of Chicago Press.

Rueda, D. (2005). Insider–outsider politics in industrialized democracies: the challenge to social democratic parties. *American Political Science Review*, *99*(01), 61–74.

Sabbath, E. L., Guevara, I. M., Glymour, M. M., & Berkman, L. F. (2015). Use of life course work–family profiles to predict mortality risk among U.S. women. *American Journal of Public Health*, *105*(4), e96–e102.

Sampson, R. J. (2012). *Great American city: Chicago and the enduring neighborhood effect*. Chicago, IL: University of Chicago Press.

Saperstein, A., & Penner, A. M. (2012). Racial fluidity and inequality in the United States. *American Journal of Sociology*, *118*(3), 676–727.

Sassen, S. (2006). *Territory, authority, rights: From medieval to global assemblages,* Princeton, NJ: Princeton University Press.

Schilt, K. (2006). Just one of the guys? How transmen make gender visible at work. *Gender and Society*, *20*(4), 465–490.

Schilt, K. (2010). *Just one of the guys? Transgender men and the persistence of gender inequality*. Chicago, IL: University of Chicago Press.

Schofer, E., & Hironaka, A. (2005). The effects of world society on environmental protection outcomes. *Social Forces*, *84*(1), 25–47.

Scruggs, L. (2004). Welfare state entitlements data set: a comparative institutional analysis of eighteen welfare states. http://cwed2.org/.

Seidman, G. W. (1999). Gendered Citizenship: South Africa's democratic transition and the construction of a gendered state. *Gender and Society*, *13*(3), 287–307. https://doi.org/10.1177/089124399013003002

Shandra, J. M., Nobles, J., London, B., & Williamson, J. B. (2004). Dependency, democracy, and infant mortality: a quantitative, cross-national analysis of less developed countries. *Social Science and Medicine, 59*(2), 321–333. https://doi.org/10.1016/j.socscimed.2003.10.022

Shostak, S., & Beckfield, J. (2015). Making a case for genetics: interdisciplinary visions and practices in the contemporary social sciences. *Advances in Medical Sociology, 16*, 95–125.

Simmons, B. A., Dobbin, F., & Garrett, G. (2008). *The Global Diffusion of Markets and Democracy.* New York, NY: Cambridge University Press.

Skocpol, T., & Amenta, E. (1986). States and social policies. *Annual Review of Sociology, 12*(1), 131–157.

Small, M. L. (2011, July 8). How to conduct a mixed methods study: Recent trends in a rapidly growing literature [review-article]. *Annual Review of Sociology, 37,* 57–86.

Smith, G. D., Shipley, M. J., & Rose, G. (1990). Magnitude and causes of socioeconomic differentials in mortality: further evidence from the Whitehall Study. *Journal of Epidemiology and Community Health, 44*(4), 265–270.

Social Security Benefit Calculator Description. (n.d.). Retrieved February 11, 2017, from https://www.ssa.gov/oact/anypia/description.html.

Somers, P., & Block, F. (2005). From poverty to perversity: Ideas, markets and institutions over 200 years of welfare debate. *American Sociological Review, 70*(3), 260–287.

Song, S., & Burgard, S. A. (2008). Social conditions and infant mortality in China: A test of the fundamental cause. California Center for Population Research. Retrieved from http://escholarship.org/uc/item/0r6938nn.pdf.

Sosnaud, B., & Beckfield, J. (2017). Trading equality for health? Social inequalities in child mortality in developing nations. *Journal of Health and Social Behavior, 58*(3), 340–356.

Star, S. L. (1999). The ethnography of infrastructure. *American Behavioral Scientist, 43*(3), 377–391. https://doi.org/10.1177/00027649921955326

Steensland, B. (2006). Cultural categories and the American welfare state: the case of guaranteed income policy. *American Journal of Sociology, 111*(5), 1273–1326.

Stimson, J. A., Mackuen, M. B., & Erikson, R. S. (1995). Dynamic representation. *American Political Science Review, 89*(3), 543–565. https://doi.org/10.2307/2082973

Stinchcombe, A. L. (1997). On the virtues of the old institutionalism. *Annual Review of Sociology*, *23*(1), 1–18. https://doi.org/10.1146/annurev.soc.23.1.1

Storeygard, A., Balk, D., Levy, M., & Deane, G. (2008). The global distribution of infant mortality: a subnational spatial view. *Population, Space and Place*, *14*(3), 209–229. https://doi.org/10.1002/psp.484

Streeck, W. (2009). *Re-forming Capitalism: Institutional Change in the German Political Economy*. Oxford, UK: Oxford University Press.

Streeck, W., & Thelen, K. A. (2005). *Beyond Continuity: Institutional Change in Advanced Political Economies*. Oxford, UK: Oxford University Press.

Stryker, R. (2013). Law and society approaches. In A. C. Wagenaar & S. C. Burris (Eds.), *Public Health Law Research: Theory and Methods* (pp. 87–108). New York, NY: Wiley.

Swiss, L. (2009). Decoupling values from action: An event-history analysis of the election of women to Parliament in the developing world, 1945–90. *International Journal of Comparative Sociology*, *50*(1), 69–95. https://doi.org/10.1177/0020715208100981

Taylor, S. E., Repetti, R. L., & Seeman, T. (1997). Health psychology: what is an unhealthy environment and how does it get under the skin? *Annual Review of Psychology*, *48*(1), 411–447.

The Macro Data Guide. (n.d.). Retrieved November 10, 2016, from http://www.nsd.uib.no/macrodataguide/index.html.

Tilly, C., (1990). *Coercion, Capital, and European States, 990–1990*. Malden, MA: Blackwell.

Timmermans, S., & Epstein, S. (2010). A world of standards but not a standard world: toward a sociology of standards and standardization. *Annual Review of Sociology*, *36*(1), 69–89. https://doi.org/10.1146/annurev.soc.012809.102629

Torres, J. M., & Waldinger, R. (2015). Civic stratification and the exclusion of undocumented immigrants from cross-border health care. *Journal of Health and Social Behavior*, *56*(4), 438–459. https://doi.org/10.1177/0022146515610617

Trinitapoli, J., & Yeatman, S. (2011). Uncertainty and fertility in a generalized AIDS epidemic. *American Sociological Review*, 76(6), 935–954.

Uggen, C., & Manza, J. (2002). Democratic contraction? Political consequences of felon disenfranchisement in the United States. *American Sociological Review*, 67(6), 777–803. https://doi.org/10.2307/3088970

US Department of Commerce, B. E. A. (n.d.). Bureau of Economic Analysis. Retrieved February 12, 2017, from https://www.bea.gov/index.htm.

van Hedel, K., Avendano, M., Berkman, L. F., Bopp, M., Deboosere, P., Lundberg, O., & Mackenbach, J. P. (2015). The contribution of national disparities to international differences in mortality between the United States and 7 European countries. *American Journal of Public Health*, 105(4), e112–e119. https://doi.org/10.2105/AJPH.2014.302344

van Hedel, K., Mejía-Guevara, I., Avendaño, M., Sabbath, E. L., Berkman, L. F., Mackenbach, J. P., & van Lenthe, F. J. (2016). Work–family trajectories and the higher cardiovascular risk of American women relative to women in 13 European countries. *American Journal of Public Health*, 106(8), 1449–1456. https://doi.org/10.2105/AJPH.2016.303264

Vandenbroucke, J. P., Broadbent, A., & Pearce, N. (2016). Causality and causal inference in epidemiology: the need for a pluralistic approach. *International Journal of Epidemiology*, 45(6), 1776–1786.

VanderWeele, T. J., Hernán, M. A., Tchetgen Tchetgen, E. J., & Robins, J. M. (2016). Re: Causality and causal inference in epidemiology: the need for a pluralistic approach. *International Journal of Epidemiology*, 45(6), 2199–2200.

Visser, J. (2011). ICTWSS: Database on institutional characteristics of trade unions, wage setting, state intervention and social pacts in 34 countries between 1960 and 2007. *Institute for Advanced Labour Studies, AIAS, University of Amsterdam, Amsterdam*. Retrieved from http://www.uva-aias.net/208.

Viterna, J. (2013). *Women in War: The Micro-processes of Mobilization in El Salvador*. New York, NY: Oxford University Press.

Viterna, J., & Robertson, C. (2015). New directions for the sociology of development. *Annual Review of Sociology*, 41, 243–269.

Walby, S. (2005). Gender mainstreaming: productive tensions in theory and practice. *Social Politics: International Studies in Gender, State and Society, 12*(3), 321–343. https://doi.org/10.1093/sp/jxi018

Weber, M. (2009). *From Max Weber: Essays in Sociology*. London, UK: Routledge.

Weed, D. L. (2016). Commentary: Causal inference in epidemiology: potential outcomes, pluralism and peer review. *International Journal of Epidemiology, 45*(6), 1838–1840.

Wendt, C., Frisina, L., & Rothgang, H. (2009). Healthcare system types: a conceptual framework for comparison. *Social Policy and Administration, 43*(1), 70–90.

Wendt, C., Grimmeisen, S., & Rothgang, H. (2005). Convergence or divergence in OECD health care systems. In B. Cantillon & I. Marx (Eds.), *International Cooperation in Social Security. How to Cope with Globalisation* (pp. 15–45). Antwerp, Belgium: Intersentia.

Western, B. (1997). *Between class and market: Postwar unionization in the capitalist democracies*. New York, NY: Cambridge University Press.

Western, B. (2006). *Punishment and inequality in America*. New York, NY: Russell Sage Foundation.

Whyte, M. K. (2005). Rethinking equality and inequality in the PRC. In *The 50th anniversary conference for the Fairbank Center for East Asian Research*. Retrieved from http://dev.wcfia.harvard.edu/sites/default/files/1068__MKW_rethinkingequality.pdf.

Whyte, M. K. (2010). Social change and the urban-rural divide in China. *The Irish Asia Strategy and Its China Relations*. Amsterdam: Rozenberg Publishers. Retrieved from http://scholar.harvard.edu/martinwhyte/files/social_change_and_the_urban-rural_divide_in_china.pdf.

Whyte, M. K., & Tsang, A. (forthcoming). China's rural-urban health gap: Paradoxical results of health insurance reforms. In Y. Li & Y. Bian (Eds.), *Social Inequalities in China*. London, UK: World Scientific and Imperial College Press.

Wigley, S., & Akkoyunlu-Wigley, A. (2011). Do electoral institutions have an impact on population health? *Public Choice, 148*(3–4), 595–610.

Wilensky, H. L. (2002). *Rich democracies: Political economy, public policy, and performance*. Berkeley and Los Angeles, CA: University of California Press.

Wilkinson, R. G., & Pickett, K. E. (2006). Income inequality and population health: a review and explanation of the evidence. *Social Science & Medicine*, 62(7), 1768–1784.

Willson, A. E., Shuey, K. M., & Elder, G. H. (2007). Cumulative advantage processes as mechanisms of inequality in life course health. *American Journal of Sociology*, 112(6), 1886–1924.

Wimmer, A., & Glick Schiller, N. (2002). Methodological nationalism and beyond: nation-state building, migration and the social sciences. *Global Networks*, 2(4), 301–334.

Woolf, S. H., & Aron, L. (2013). *U.S. Health in International Perspective: Shorter Lives, Poorer Health*. Washington, DC: National Academies Press.

Xie, Y. (2013). Population heterogeneity and causal inference. *Proceedings of the National Academy of Sciences*, 110(16), 6262–6268. https://doi.org/10.1073/pnas.1303102110

Zimmerman, F. J. (2008). A commentary on 'Neo-materialist theory and the temporal relationship between income inequality and longevity change'. *Social Science & Medicine*, 66(9), 1882–1894.

INDEX